the ILLUSION of PSYCHOTHERAPY

William M. Epstein

The Illusion of Psychotherapy

Routledge
Taylor & Francis Group
LONDON AND NEW YORK

First published 1995 by Transaction Publishers

2 Park Square, Milton Park, Abingdon, Oxfordshire OX14 4RN
711 Third Avenue, New York, NY 10017

Routledge is an imprint of the Taylor & Francis Group, an informa business

First issued in paperback 2018

Library of Congress Catalog Number: 95-5273

Library of Congress Cataloging-in-Publication Data

Epstein, William M., 1944-
The illusion of psychotherapy / William M. Epstein.
p. cm.
Includes bibliographical references and index.
ISBN 1-56000-215-8
1. Psychotherapy—Evaluation. 2. Social problems. 3. Psychotherapy—Political aspects. 4. Social control. 5. Ideology. 6. United States—Social policy—1980-1993. I. Title.
RC480.5.E66 1995
616.89'14—dc20 95-5273
CIP

ISBN 13: 978-1-56000-215-4 (hbk)
ISBN 13: 978-1-138-51611-3 (pbk)

Laura, Peter, Matthew

Contents

Preface

No style of clinical wisdom has translated into any systematic and credible evidence that psychotherapy is effective in handling personal or social problems. The theories that underpin clinical practice remain speculative while their influence over social policy is more ideological than scientific. Psychotherapists and their credulous patients are welcome to the special preserve of their pleas that therapy is a heroic pursuit of an elusive and personal epiphany that transcends rigorous standards of proof. But a skeptical public and its government are better served by an attachment to tangible evidence of outcomes.

I have chosen to evaluate psychotherapy against its claims to remedy personal dysfunctions and their consequent social problems. These claims should be measured as objective changes in the behaviors associated with the problems. This analysis is admittedly limited to the mundane, the question of whether psychotherapy is effective against a variety of unwanted human behaviors such as drug addiction and depression.

I cannot pretend to a deep understanding of the human soul or human behavior. The sublime in human experience may simply be beyond the possibility of graphic proof. It may also be irrelevant to social problems and the public policy-making process.

Through years of attention to the many claims that social problems can be inexpensively resolved, and frequently through one sort of psychotherapy or another, I have come in the end to believe in money as the essential element of a cure for what ails contemporary America with the same intensity that the Ancient Mariner believed in fresh water as a cure for thirst. Within the limitations imposed by concreteness and specificity, I have constructed a sense of the nation's social problems that speaks directly to the inadequacies of its central social institutions: families, communities, education, jobs, and so forth.

Social problems emerge by and large because many people are brought up in deficient families; live in perilous, inattentive communities; lack education and jobs; have no routes out of poverty; and are exposed to unreasonable and unrelenting risks to their physical and mental health. These institutional deficiencies are measurable. Moreover, it is a central tenet of modern liberal democracy that most deficiencies are possible to remedy through a series of surrogate arrangements—human services.

This position is inevitably unpopular since it requires massive new resources or the extensive redistribution of existing resources. Both strategies seem unlikely, a failure of purpose that impedes progress against social problems. I hope that this book draws attention back to the social policy option of pursuing basic cultural sufficiency. This implies greater social equality as opposed to its mockery in policies that seek to legitimize the nation's telling inequalities as cultural diversity.

Partial solutions are no solution at all. While comprehensive reform is not yet politically feasible, the direction of the United States encourages longer-range thinking in anticipation of a time when bolder ideas may be politically acceptable. Wisdom may lie along the line of providing all Americans with a decent experience in their own culture. This requires adequate participation in basic American institutions: family, community, school, work, and so forth. The extent of our problems—and poverty is just one of them—reflects the degree to which deficits in basic social institutions have been tolerated.

At least one special relationship with at least one responsible adult; literacy and civility; career training; a job with opportunities for retraining and upgrading; medical security; financial security for old age; and so forth would operationalize cultural sufficiency. These very basic sorts of things have been lacking while psychotherapy and other forms of socially therapeutic interventions have not provided an adequate substitute. The constant choice of psychotherapy and social therapeutics generally diverts recurrent impulses to address poverty into inexpensive but ineffective strategies.

There is something amiss with our intellectual life. For many years now, commentary on social welfare has centered on the narrow problems of the federal budget deficit, ignoring growing social needs and the problems caused by large social equalities in the United States. The literature of psychotherapy has not played an independent scientific role in this debate nor a role on behalf of those in need. Unfortunately, it has become a pawn in social dialectics.

Over the years I have accumulated an intellectual debt to J. R. Ravetz, particularly for his book *Scientific Knowledge and Its Social Problems,* that I have only acknowledged indirectly through quotations and citations in my papers. Unlike the many postmodernists, he has recognized the social intrusions into science without capitulating to the whimsy that social reality is only a product of social will or that science and objectivity are impossible pursuits. His wonderful good humor and his grand erudition have inspired me.

A number of people patiently read through drafts and offered thoughtful and focused comments. The book is a better work for the help of Marvin Bloom, Laura Epstein, Paul M. Epstein, Irving Louis Horowitz, Joyce Lai Mah, Theo Manschreck, Brij Mohan, Robert Morris, Douglas R. Imig, Gage W. Chapel, Gerald Rubin, and Linda Santangelo. I am particularly grateful for the intelligence and careful work of my research assistants—Susan Gunn, Dorothea S. Arin, Pamela Rucker-Larmouth, and Janie Ostlund. While my analyses and insights owe much to the comments of editors, readers, reviewers, and assistants, I will not share the distinction of my errors with anyone.

I am also thankful for financial support and encouragement from David N. McNelis, Associate Vice President for Research at the University of Nevada, Las Vegas.

Acknowledgments

Occasional portions of various chapters—the descriptions of Miller et al. 1989, Kazdin 1989, Smith, Glass, and Miller 1980, and the summary of the other meta-analyses—are taken from W. M. Epstein 1993.

1

Introduction

"It takes a certain moral courage to accept the message of scientific ignorance and all that it implies."

—R. C. Lewontin

The shelf is bare on which credible proof of the effectiveness of psychotherapy should be accumulating. For more than fifty years, the field of psychotherapy has accepted at least the desirability of social science methods in testing its effectiveness. Yet, despite its avowed commitments, the field has routinely defied standard procedures of clinical proof. Today there is not one credible study conforming to the basic rules of objective proof that testifies to the effectiveness of any psychotherapeutic treatment. To the contrary, the manifest biases of the research, as well as systematic inferences of client deterioration, suggest grounds on which to assume the actual ineffectiveness and possible harm of psychotherapy—not just the indeterminacy of its benefits.

If society responded rationally to the demonstrated weaknesses of psychotherapy, then the field would be in decline. Yet, in spite of the thoroughgoing absence of credible tests of its effectiveness—and even in light of the probability of its ineffectiveness and harm—psychotherapy, and social therapeutics generally, steadfastly remain immensely popular both as treatments for a variety of personal and social problems and as justifications for minimal and routinely ineffective social interventions. Psychotherapy plays a political role that transcends its defining production functions to provide personal services and to measure the effects of those services against personal and social standards of prevention, cure, and rehabilitation.

The broader notion of social therapeutics encapsulates the metaphor of medicine as preventative vaccine and curative pill for both personal and societal ills. Social therapy, relying upon the belief that personal behavior can be purposively changed, underpins contemporary social policy in the United States as well as other modern industrial nations. An immense array of social services and opportunities are provided to the American public—education, medical and mental health care, job preparation, child foster care and protective services, corrections, and drug and alcohol rehabilitation are a few examples—and justified by the notion that they are in a variety of ways therapeutic, that is, that their provision either enhances life or prevents its deterioration. Even the social insurances—unemployment insurance and Old Age, Survivors, Disability, and Health Insurance (OASDHI)—can be interpreted in the context of America's social dialectics of therapy as treatments for the risks of poverty, disability, and ill health.

Prevention and social rehabilitation are deeply valued in the American culture. Both notions assume that human behavior is relatively malleable and that planful action, usually in the form of rational science, is capable of guiding steps to prevent and to treat social and personal problems. Psychotherapy is perhaps the most refined expression and the most widely accepted discipline of social therapeutics. In its many forms it has been prescribed for the range of psychiatric and personal problems that underpin social problems and personal distress. Moreover, psychotherapy has been relied on by Becker and by Rieff, as two conventional examples, and in the extremes even by many liberationist doctrines as a language and as a technique to provide insight and correct thought.

As political responses to personal distress, social services based upon psychotherapy and social therapeutics constitute conditions of citizenship in the modern state. However, social therapeutics, and psychotherapy in particular, are more than a series of specific personal interventions. The characteristics of therapeutics, elaborated within the long tradition of western socialization, also comprise a powerful social and political ideology.

The ideology of therapy expresses itself through a series of myths that define an individual's social and personal responsibilities and the obligations of society to its members. The factual content of the myths is less pertinent than their convincing ability to convey decisive metaphors of deep cultural values. In almost feudal fashion, the decisive metaphors embody the expectations of the social contract that entitles a citizen to relief of distress and obligates the society to provide specific material responses. These expectations, even when uncodified in public statutes, reside within a culture as powerful motivators that, when unfulfilled, create a deep sense of wrong and injustice.

The prescription in many psychotherapies for the patient's personal role in remedying his or her distress, that is, "to take charge of one's own life"—expressing the metaphors of independence, free will, and personal autonomy—reinforces the cherished cultural value of personal responsibility. This value is pressed without regard to the factual content of the presenting problem, that is, to the reality of whether it is feasible or desirable or, indeed, even therapeutic for the patient to accept personal responsibility. The facts of psychotherapy as a rational clinical intervention relate to the actual possibility of an individual patient's ability to take responsibility for specific behaviors and the determination of ethical responsibility for the presenting problem, that is, whether the society or the individual caused the problem and whether the patient is capable of resolving the problem without utilizing more material resources in addition to his or her own personal will. The metaphor of personal responsibility is consciously chosen over a metaphor of social causation and social responsibility that may also entail an obligation for more material remedies than the customarily verbal interchange between a trained psychotherapist and a patient.

Ideally, the metaphor of therapy should coincide with the reality of its programmatic usefulness. However, the metaphoric value of therapy as social ideology can be separated from its clinical functions. Indeed, it can exist without a true clinical function, purveying propagandistic metaphors that misrepresent both the interests and the conditions of the intended audience, including patients.

The expressive arts—literature, the visual arts, and so forth—subjectively package social morality in a variety of forms that sanction specific relations among people, defining both their appropriate roles in specific circumstances and the behaviors that can be expected to be censured or rewarded. The social sciences—the home disciplines for social therapeutics and psychotherapy and the source of their authority—also perform functions that are similar to the expressive arts since they do not contrive themselves from aprioristic assumptions in an acultural vacuum. The social sciences carry the normative weight of particular institutions and objectives. Yet, even while interpretive, the social sciences distinguish themselves from the expressive arts by tying themselves to the traditional practice of the standard sciences through a commitment to the logic of objectivity and the canons of controlled, prospective experimentation.

The social sciences attempt to objectively handle a variety of powerful metaphoric abstractions: class, race, status, prestige, deprivation, prevention, cure, treatment, and so forth. The metaphors of the social sciences, passionately accepted as the terms of modern discourse, seem to approximate the graphicness of material possessions. Indeed, the expressive arts have frequently performed the journalism of the social sciences.

The social sciences are dedicated to provide the civic culture with the systematic, credible, and authoritative information that underpins democratic decision making. The performance of the social sciences implies a pact between the citizenry and its intellectual elite to fairly monitor the culture's promises to fulfill its obligations. When therapy is successful, the implicit pact is fulfilled between the suffering patient and the culture. However, when therapy is not successful, that is, when the therapeutic intervention is insufficient to relieve the citizen's distress and when no other remedy is provided, then therapy constitutes denial of a citizen's grievance or, in the case of sanctioned behaviors such as criminality, the denial of the society's legitimate interests.

Furthermore, when therapy is unsuccessful, the refusal to acknowledge its failure subverts the basic social process of democratic policy making by withholding from the society important information about the depth of its problems and the futility of its current remedies. Nevertheless, the illusion of effectiveness may be useful for a culture that wishes to deny its problems or to ignore the needs of its citizens. The illusion of successful therapy tends to diminish dissent, reconciling complaint with social response. Strong incentives to deny more thoroughgoing responses to social complaints can create powerful incentives to endorse the appearance of effectiveness. Acting through material rewards and social prestige, the motives to satisfy political orthodoxy may distort the commitments of a professional subcommunity.

Psychotherapy covers a range of interventions. Generally, the variety of psychotherapies fall between two types: (1) cognitive approaches, largely inspired by Freudian, insight, and humanistic schools that employ rational induction as a primary technique; and (2) behavioral approaches growing out of psychological learning theory that employ a variety of conditioning schemes to modify specific dysfunctional behaviors. While Beck has developed a specific course of treatment that is called *cognitive therapy,* or sometimes *cognitive behavioral therapy,* the concept is more generic. Cognitive therapy's core assumption—that cognitions precede behavior and that by changing cognitions, behavior will change—is also shared by a variety of schools (e.g., psychodynamic, interpersonal, and strategic), which each emphasize different durations, intensities, and targets of intervention. All of the cognitive therapies share a common treatment strategy; each school maintains that conscious reasoning and verbal interaction between the therapist and the patient constitute the heart of the healing process.

In contrast, behavioral therapies focuses principally on the behaviors that are the symptoms of mental illness, distress, and otherwise dysfunctional behavior. Behavioral approaches diminish the importance of self-reflection and emphasize the external conditions that account for the patient's learned dysfunctions. Behavioral therapy assumes that the same processes—classical and operant conditioning—that account for the persistence of inappropriate learned behavior can be modified to encourage the patient to learn more acceptable and satisfying behaviors. Behavioral techniques attempt to change the reinforcing conditions that explain the persistence of the patient's problems. These interventions cover an enormous range: graduated exposure, flooding, token economies, skills training, biofeedback, relaxation techniques, and others.

In spite of their formal differences, the overwhelming majority of psychotherapies share certain similarities. Psychotherapy is typically a process of interaction between a therapist with training in psychiatry, psychology, social work, or counseling, and a patient with a problem. The patient can receive the therapy individually, in a group, or in a family. The psychotherapeutic session is customarily confined to an office or hospital; patients are rarely, if ever, seen in their homes or in their own social environments. Apart from psychoanalysis, the Freudian inspiration for psychotherapy, therapy typically lasts less than one year, and in recent times, the customary course of therapy is completed within a few months. In contrast to biological therapies (e.g., drug therapy and shock therapy), psychotherapy for mental and social problems involves only verbal or other symbolic interventions.

In sum, psychotherapy promises to change personally problematic behaviors that are frequently associated with social problems through relatively inexpensive, short-term, and socially compatible processes. This is an immensely attractive strategy for a society that is reluctant to allocate substantial funds to address its problems. If it were effective, then psychotherapy would offer efficient, low-cost remedies. Yet, even apart from the issue of its effectiveness, psychotherapy still provides a useful vehicle to proselytize the ideology of social efficiency in evading more disruptive and expensive approaches to social problems in the United States.

The Privileged Position of Psychotherapy

The political constituency for the therapeutic myth transcends the community of therapeutic professions and the human potential movement whose members skirt the margins of bogus science and faith healing in pursuing visionary, improbable solutions to social problems. The ideology of therapeutics is also consistent with a conservative social ideology that is unwilling to accept broad-based social expenditures to provide greater social equality through government action. Indeed, the therapeutic ideology amasses its support through paradoxical promises for socially efficient remedies, both the quaint expectation of rationalistic solutions to deep social distress and the promise to do so inexpensively, that is, without deep public expenditures and consequently without major disruptions of society.

The large political constituency that is animated by socially efficient possibilities suffers little opposition. Current American politics are undisturbed by proposals for overhauls of its social welfare system. The difficulty of effecting even modest increases in entitlements for education, medical coverage, welfare, child care, unemployment protection, job training and retraining, community safety, and other institutions of the American culture goes far to explain the persistence of therapeutics, a social welfare strategy that denies the necessity of compensating for prior social deprivations.

Not surprisingly, the effectiveness of psychotherapy is as widely accepted outside of the psychotherapeutic community as within its own circle of practitioners and researchers. The few empirically grounded skeptics (Eysenck, Rachman, Bergin, and others who are discussed in subsequent chapters) prior to the 1980 publication of *The Benefits of Psychotherapy* and the smaller number afterwards such as Kline (1988),

Prioleau, Murdock, and Brody (1983), and Dawes (1994) constitute a small and ineffectual critical tradition within the field that has largely been ignored by the culture. Psychotherapy has customarily been treated with soft hands even by recent critics who have rigorously condemned a variety of bogus techniques to improve human performance and reduce psychic distress.

An important study, conducted on behalf of the United States Army by the National Academy of Sciences, analyzed both mainstream and parapsychological performance enhancement techniques; but it ignored psychotherapy. Nevertheless, their review and the assumptions of their analysis offer a model for evaluating psychotherapy itself:

> Implementation of an enhancement technique, in the committee's view, should depend on two general kinds, or levels, of evaluation. The first examines primarily the scientific justification for the effectiveness of the technique and the potential of the technique for improving performance in practice. The second kind examines field tests of a pilot program incorporating the technique to determine how feasible it is and to what extent it brings about effects that Army officials consider useful. (Druckman and Swets 1988, 25)

Their review found limited evidence in support of improving motor skills and stress management. Yet the committee found no scientific evidence, but a lot of questionable and bogus data, in support of learning during sleep, accelerated learning, altering mental states, influence strategies, group cohesion, and parapsychological phenomena. Moreover, their cautious report identified very little support in the vast specialized literature for the effectiveness of any performance enhancement technique and even fewer definitive studies of scientific merit. In spite of decades of extensive public support, the scientific literature covering performance enhancement techniques failed to accumulate a credible body of research. While the United States Army could take comfort that its own training methods were on track, the social sciences and the social services themselves could take little pride in the quality of their research.

Specht (1990), in discussing the utility for social work of what he terms popular psychotherapy, has been curiously protective of psychotherapy and psychoanalysis.

> Popular psychotherapy, as distinct from psychoanalytically oriented therapy, does not date back to Freud. Rather, its historical roots lie in great social movements of early-nineteenth-century America, beginning in approximately the 1830's. That is, psychotherapy today (both the serious and the "flaky") is primarily not Freudian.

> Its origins are more American than Austrian; currently it is more humanistically oriented than it is psychoanalytic. (350)

He is derisive of the popular psychotherapies, "one of the major battalions in the armies of the secular priesthood to carry forth the tenets of the church of individual repair" (Specht 1990, 353). Specht presumably feels that the designer therapies—Freudian psychoanalysis and the derivative psychotherapies—have earned greater esteem for their success at "resocialization and restoration" (Specht 1990, 354). Nevertheless, he offers no evidence of effectiveness to exempt them from his scorn for the popular therapies. Apparently, rationalistic, university-based psychotherapy confers greater status on social work than would the less institutionalized popular therapies even while the curative powers of both types may be equally negligible. Specht's argument is typical both of the protection given to psychotherapy and the intuitive grounds on which its effectiveness is applauded.

Kaminer's (1992) well-received book reached more deeply into the popular therapies, in particular, self-help and personal improvement regimens, and ended up debunking them all. While her treatment was journalistic, lacking any systematic attempt to measure their effectiveness, her conclusions underlined their unfulfilled promises and the Elmer Gantry rapacity of the self-help entrepreneurs.

> For all their talk about intuitive, "feeling realities," experts rely on readers' willingness to surrender not just rationality but intuition, by which they might lead themselves to unsuspected places. Experts exalt intuition, but they don't actually value it. How could they? It would threaten their business much more than intellectualism ever has or could. (165)

Her pointed discussion takes to task programs based upon "popular notions of self-actualization and self-effacement" for creating the very dependency they decry by demanding cultlike obedience, conformity, and unquestioning belief. Yet in the end, Kaminer too exempts psychotherapy and psychotherapists from her contempt, holding them safe from the shared judgment that psychotherapy, as much as self-help regimens, may impose a chain hotel personality on its patients through similarly cultish demands for unthinking devotion.

Gross's (1978) earlier critique of psychotherapy anticipated Kaminer's work. Gross examined the religious nature of psychotherapy and its use as social ritual. Yet he and Kaminer, and the small amount of critical literature in the field that discusses the effectiveness of its outcomes, failed to identify the social motives and political conditions that sustain both the popular and the sublime psychotherapies.

The marketplace for unconventional therapy is immense. Eisenberg and his associates, reporting in *The New England Journal of Medicine* (Eisenberg et al. 1993), surveyed 1,539 respondents to measure their use, over the previous twelve months, of a variety of unconventional therapies: relaxation techniques, chiropractic, massage, imagery, spiritual healing, commercial weight-loss programs, lifestyle diets (e.g., macrobiotics), herbal medicine, megavitamin therapy, self-help groups, energy healing, biofeedback, hypnosis, homeopathy, acupuncture, and folk remedies. They found that 34 percent of all respondents reported the use of at least one of these therapies. Thirty six percent of these respondents (and therefore about 12 percent of all respondents) reported that they had actually seen a provider of an unconventional therapy, averaging nineteen visits to these providers over the previous twelve months.

The Eisenberg study did not include psychotherapy as an alternative therapy apparently because it is "in conformity with the standards of the medical community" and, therefore, constitutes mainline scientific practice. However, the assumed conformity of psychotherapy with standard medical research implies only customary acceptance and not the presence of any evidence that distinguishes the effectiveness of psychotherapy from unorthodox, alternative techniques of putative value.

Virtually indistinguishable from the typical self-help manuals of Specht's popular therapies or even the cultish publications of many alternative therapies, a recent book by Hillman and Ventura (1992), who are therapists themselves, is characteristic of the psychotherapy literature that finds its way to a nonprofessional public. Hillman and Ventura write in an intensely self-absorbed style, through a series of notes and dialogues between the two authors. Isolated within the drama of therapy and patients, their criticism of the field rests not on its questionable effectiveness but on its parochialism, its timidity in avoiding the problems of the world.

The intellectual community has largely accepted the field's prevailing judgment of itself: psychotherapy has made important progress over the past few decades as a reputable scientific discipline in developing effective clinical remedies for mental illness. While the different psychotherapies, at times, go after each other's throats, the issues of psychotherapy's fundamental effectiveness infrequently enter the public debate over social policy. Indeed, these questions have been raised by only a few persistent critics, notably Eysenck and Rachman.

Many of the field's deepest critics, such as Rieff and Szasz, frequently indict the field more for its complicity in illegitimate social control and in medical imperialism than for its defects as clinical science. Indeed, much of the criticism of psychotherapy assumes its clinical effectiveness. This assumption of effectiveness is frequently a necessary component of the criticisms on other grounds; an argument against a straw man is pointless and the drama of the criticism is heightened by the general perception of the field's clinical power. In any event, many critics, while troubled over the field's probity or weak methodologies or both, seem to accept the ability of psychotherapy to achieve at least some of its clinical goals.[1]

Nevertheless, moral speculations over the social impact of psychotherapy carry greater weight to the extent to which the field flourishes *without* a demonstrable ability to treat mental illness.[2] If psychotherapy does not have an ability to address emotional and mental problems, and if it is routinely harmful, then its ceremonial functions—the social influence of psychotherapy exercised as myth and its political utility—stand out boldly to explain its persistence and commercial success. The possibility of a barren production function in treating mental illness actually reinforces Szasz's concern that psychotherapy principally fulfills an ideological function and perhaps even the one he identifies of justifying coercion and circumscribing liberty.

The largest amount of successful criticism of the field's clinical effectiveness has centered on the scientific inadequacies of Freudian psychoanalysis and of Freud as a scientist. Except for a small group of committed psychoanalysts, the larger field of psychotherapy customarily acknowledges many of the deficiencies of the founder's theory and practice while still insisting that it has progressed since Freud, achieving major advances in the treatment of mental and emotional problems through the application of a rigorous clinical science. However, the same reservations that seem to be tipping critical opinion out of favor with extended psychoanalysis are equally applicable to the entire field of psychotherapy and even to the domain of social therapeutics.

Grunbaum (1984) and Hook (1959), among others, shredded the rational pretenses of psychoanalytic psychotherapy, that is, psychoanalysis, as a modern scientific discipline, in the process reducing the stature of Freud as a scientist. Grunbaum provided a warrant for experimental tests of psychoanalysis' effectiveness (1984). He argued that scientific procedures were required to test the standing of psychoanalysis as a clinically responsible intervention. He rejected the ability of hermeneutic techniques—"empathy and intuitive self-evidence"—and other evidence generated by patients "from the couch" (from introspective reports and projective techniques such as free association) to provide accurate data to test the effectiveness of the field or the viability of its theories.

Grunbaum (1984) argued that Freudian psychoanalysis was in the end amenable to scientific testing at least in principle even while it had escaped systematic scrutiny in fact. Ernest Nagel (among others, in Hook 1959) denied psychoanalytic theory even this much. In contrast to Grunbaum (1984), he claimed that psychoanalysis is self-certifying and, thus, fails to define either theoretical concepts that are falsifiable or the conditions under which they could be tested, that is, specific test conditions which if met would prove the theory true and if not met would prove the theory false. In Nagel's sense (Hook 1959), psychoanalytic theory fails to make specific predictions that can be empirically checked.

Yet, even if psychoanalytic theory is unavailable for direct verification, its clinical practice still can be treated as a "black box" whose impacts can be measured without knowing how they are produced. With appropriate controls and other methodological safeguards in place—randomized controlled clinical trials—the status of patients before therapy can be compared with their status after therapy. While a "black box" procedure can not throw light on the causes of specific outcomes, it can measure the clinical effectiveness of an intervention.

Grunbaum (1984) underscored the need for objective tests, that is, "extra-clinical studies," of psychoanalysis' effectiveness. He rejected Freud's notion that psychoanalytic theory could be adequately tested by the "consilience" of psychohistorical information drawn from the patient by the therapist through a variety of psychoanalytic techniques. Grunbaum (1984) argued that an apparent coherence could be induced by the analyst's influence over the patient—the patient's susceptibility to the analyst's suggestions—in such a way that the analyst's theory of the patient's problems would supplant the patient's report of his actual history. This is precisely the source of the skepticism that questions the accuracy of adult recollections of their allegedly repressed memories of childhood incest. The analyst's influence over the patient, together with the analyst's professional stake in particular outcomes, suggested the need for independent judges and for objective behavior measures to assess the effects of psychotherapy.

The potential bias of therapists—or any caregiver—in assessing their own effectiveness is precisely the reason that credible clinical research requires reliable, objective procedures to assess outcomes. Patient self-reports are not credible sources of objective fact, even about the patient's own behaviors. Moreover, the suggestibility of patients becomes a pointed issue when the researcher is a strong advocate of the techniques being evaluated and when his or her expectancies for particular outcomes can be transmitted even unwittingly to his research subjects.

Still, Grunbaum (1984) never demonstrated that analysts actually transmitted their biases to their patients, nor that the patient's self-reports were faulty.[3] But he did not need to prove the existence of these biases in order to condemn research that relied upon potentially biased data or that failed to implement appropriate safeguards against bias. Nevertheless, others have documented powerful researcher expectancy biases in psychological research (Rosenthal and Rubin 1978).

Grunbaum (1984) argued tacitly from the premise that the burden to prove the effectiveness of psychoanalysis rested firmly on the shoulders of the field and that it had still not proven its clinical value. He dismissed the value of its outcome literature, anticipating the euphemistic observation that psychoanalysts "are not inclined to perform research studies" (American Psychiatric Association 1989, 1833). A portion of that burden of proof entailed the credible measurement of outcomes, which in turn implied "extra-clinical" evaluations based upon neutrally validated changes in patient behaviors and not upon the analyst's report of his or her own progress nor the patient's testimonials to the benefits of psychoanalysis.

Grunbaum's (1984) insistence on the application of scientific standards to the psychoanalytic enterprise is given greater force when the analyst and psychoanalytic theory are interpreted as mediating the broader culture. This extended interpretation in which therapists act as the agents of the culture suggests that a false "consilience" of evidence and the distortion of research generally are more than the aberrant results of a similarly motivated group of people sharing similar biases: analysts pursuing professional advancement and social prestige on the basis of their ability to cure psychic distress. Rather, the shaping of professional truths is one of the customary routes through which a dominant culture nourishes compatible ideology by imposing its preferences on one of its component institutions. The practice of a politically sensitive psychotherapy routinely distorts the objectivity of its own research in pursuit of social approval and rewards. The culture itself, selectively rewarding the compatible expectancy biases of therapists, creates myths of acceptable social behavior. Porous research becomes politically useful. In this way, the field of psychotherapy feeds off of political preferences for socially efficient interventions.

These social motives act throughout the geography of a homogeneous and highly centralized society such as the United States. The unseen hand of culture perfuses apparently separate and independent research activities, orchestrating each other's corroborating distortions through vulnerable methodologies. Without appropriate methodological safeguards against the pitfalls of bias, the replication of experiments becomes politically obsequious. Prevailing social values, diffused by faulty science, traps the practice of psychotherapy. This is the sort of social process that endorses the plausibility of Rieff's (1966) criticisms: although psychotherapy was initially inspired as a release from the constraining orthodoxies of culture, the practice of psychotherapy has become co-opted as one of its agents of illegitimate control.

Curiously, Grunbaum's (1984) argument seemed to be fresh at least for the field of psychoanalysis as recently as the 1980s. The psychoanalytic subcommunity itself, as well as the broader society, apparently needed to be reminded that the theory and the practice of psychoanalysis still failed to conform to even rudimentary rules of scientific proof. Grunbaum (1984) was not simply pressing against an intellectual recalcitrance in psychoanalysis, and perhaps its favored social position, but also against a broader intellectual fashion that favored weak methodologies, such as Habermas's hermeneutics, over objective science. Grunbaum refused to grant psychoanalysis either permission to swim in a soup of postmodern subjectivity or a waiver from the logic of the natural sciences in testing its outcomes.

Even as late as 1994 prominent psychotherapists were still arguing that psychoanalysis was an effective intervention, in spite of their very grudging acknowledgment of Freudian therapy's imperfections, and still offering proofs of its effectiveness that were based upon case studies and evidence that had accrued from their own private practices (*New York Review* 1994). In response to Crews's (1993) summary of the clinical and theoretical pitfalls of psychoanalysis and the shortcomings of Freud, leading psychoanalysts, including many holding positions in medical schools and other academic departments, protested that the criticisms were off the mark; indifferent to the progress of contemporary practice; only ad hominem rebukes to Freud and not indictments of psychoanalysis itself; ignorant of Freud's true methods; and naive (*New York Review* 1994).

> Because [Crews] describes some definitely "unscientific" aspects in the history of psychoanalysis, it implies that current practice is still, wild, capricious, and self-serving on the part of analysts. (Olds in *New York Review* 1994, 35)
>
> I am a member of a psychoanalytic study group.... Over the years our group...has repeatedly discussed these same issues, questioning the matter of proof.... But as the article goes on an intemperate note enters into the argument, an angry and ad hominem note. (Peyser in *New York Review* 1994, 34)
>
> For...symptom neuroses and personality disorders that impair the individual's ability to enjoy a loving relation with another person, or to apply himself successfully to any vocation or to escape from a prevailing self-defeating tendency...psychotherapies are prescribed. The extraordinary rates of success advertised by the practitioners [of various psychotherapies] are probably exaggerated but there is no doubt that the treatment does succeed in many instances. However, for the treatment of other neuroses and the personality disorders, a patient oriented psychotherapy is required. (Ostrow in *New York Review* 1994)
>
> [Crews] is clearly a man who reads and writes a lot about psychoanalysis, but there is no evidence that he has knowledge of studies on the comparison of the efficacy of psychoanalysis with other forms of psychotherapy. (Luborsky in *New York Review* 1994)

In responding to Crews, only Luborsky offered systematic evidence—a few summaries of research—that psychoanalysis is as effective as other psychotherapies. Moreover, he claimed that "the evidence is overwhelming, in fact, that these different forms of psychotherapy produce very meaningful benefits for the majority of patients" (Luborsky in the *New York Review* 1994, 37).

Contrary to Luborsky's (*New York Review* 1994) claims, there is in fact no credible evidence to support the fundamental effectiveness of either psychoanalysis or psychotherapy while the research that compares psychoanalysis with other therapies is also fundamentally flawed. Luborsky's (*New York Review* 1994) cited summaries, their base of primary clinical studies, and the rest of the field's evidence for its effectiveness (discussed in later chapters) are bulk-cargo empiricism, not credible science. Luborsky's recent evidence, which he claims represents important methodological progress for the field, is in the end no more believable than the unverified personal testimonies of psychoanalysts and the reports of their gullible patients. While draped in the robes of science the contemporary research in psychotherapy suffers the same pitfalls as the psychoanalytic research, resisting the spirit of science and its required methods.

Still, Crews (1993) could have profitably extended his observations; his criticism of psychoanalysis for its rudimentary failure at the enterprise of science is generally applicable to all of psychotherapy and social therapeutics. It is a tribute to the culture's enduring affection for even the psychoanalytic form of therapy that comfortable practices are still possible for seemingly interminable courses of treatment and that professional opinion still relies on evidence from the couch and on therapists' assessments of their own effectiveness.

The apparent decline in extended psychoanalysis over the past years has not occurred because of attenuated public or professional enthusiasms. Rather, insurance companies have refused to underwrite questionable treatments that go on for years while the field itself has produced short-term designer substitutes for the full course of psychoanalysis. Unfortunately, managed care insurance schemes in the pursuit of greater business profits seem only to have reduced the available funds to care for the mentally ill. Neglect seems to have been made more efficient. Neither Grunbaum (1984), Hook (1959), Kurzweil (1989), Roazan (1990), Rosen (1968), nor Crews (1993) extended their arguments past psychoanalysis to psychotherapy generally. It is not clear that they directly addressed the issue of psychoanalysis' effectiveness, preferring to focus on epistemology, history, conflict between divergent schools, and its meaning as social ideology and not on the facts of its clinical performance. Yet, even in the few instances when the field's effectiveness is questioned (for example, Klerman 1983, 1986, 1990), there is little appreciation for the possibility that its very weaknesses may be structural and socially useful and not simply the customary products of professional self-protectiveness.

The persistence of the field may have little to do with either its putative clinical value or its institutional strength, which may itself be derivative. Rather, the field probably persists largely because it creates mythic support for contemporary social preferences. This implies that the central function of psychotherapy is to facilitate dominant cultural values, not to pursue a science of treatment. In place of its ostensible attachment to rational proof and its birth within a scientific incubator, psychotherapy has emerged as a postmodern profession—an expression of politically convenient myths that are facilitated by weak methodologies of proof—and not simply as a profession in the postmodern era.

Psychotherapy and Science

Ironically, even while the field may flourish because of porous tests of its own effectiveness, psychotherapy has accepted at least formally the canon of science in order to establish its professional standing. The scientific cachet is important to elevate psychotherapy over quackery and to legitimize its role in society alongside of medicine and engineering.

The Benefits of Psychotherapy (Smith, Glass, and Miller 1980) has become a citation classic attesting to the field's effectiveness. It systematically demolished resistance to the scientific evaluation of psychotherapy arguing that rigorous, objective scrutiny of its effects are possible and, therefore, that psychotherapy is within "the realm of experimental scientific study" (Smith, Glass, and Miller 1980, 29). This position acknowledges that psychotherapy is not simply an ineffable art form, but that its outcomes, and usually its processes as well, can be defined objectively and measured quantitatively. Moreover, the authors also pointed out that randomized control groups are ethical and practical and that the effectiveness of psychotherapy and its social utility are legitimate issues for research and not simply articles of faith.

Yet, the Smith, Glass, and Miller (1980) evaluation failed to fulfill its high-minded commitment to scientific rigor in the substance of its analysis. Nevertheless, they underscored an important procedural point: the burden to prove the value of psychotherapy lies on the shoulders of the therapeutic community, not on the shoulders of the skeptic. As in medicine and pharmacology, the proponent of a cure carries the onus of proof that it is safe and effective. However, unlike pharmacological research that must conform with the methodological rigors mandated by the United States Food and Drug Administration, the psychotherapy community is free to adopt a far more compliant standard of proof.

The traditional acceptance of psychotherapy may provide social protection and an inertial sense of value, but it has no standing either ethically or logically in establishing the effectiveness of an intervention. Yet, the embeddedness of any social behavior—the popularity of psychotherapy as one example—certainly impedes rigorous evaluation and, consequently, the possibility of more effective substitutes.

Precisely the same sort of tough scrutiny that the United States Army purchased from the National Academy of Sciences is appropriate to apply to psychotherapy. On the face of it there is no essential difference in either form or purpose between psychotherapy on the one hand and alternative therapies, self-help programs, and popular psychotherapies on the other. The notion that psychotherapy enjoys an aristocratic ancestry in learning theory while the popular therapies suffer their parentage from devotional and inspirational works does not condone a lenient and gullible acceptance of psychotherapy's promises. To the contrary, the similarly cultish nature of psychotherapeutic practice and transcendental meditation, as one example, should raise a common set of suspicions.

The rigorous evaluation of psychotherapeutic practice entails the application of a particular methodology—randomized placebo-controlled trials (RPCT). This methodology is commonly acknowledged as the definitive investigatory tool of science for clinical practice generally. RPCTs are feasible, ethical, and legal. Unfortunately, they are also very expensive.

Definitive tests discipline the entire scholarly enterprise. When a field accepts this discipline, all of its research activities—initial observations, instrument construction, exploratory, descriptive, and epidemiological studies, and pilot tests—build toward a critical demonstration of effectiveness. Without the necessity to face a rigorous trial of its effectiveness, a field's research turns softly obedient to organizational and political imperatives.

RPCTs also imply prospective experimentation, a fair test to assess the effectiveness of a therapy. Historical data from the existing records of different therapies cannot assure that the data was collected in a neutral or comparable way, that the study's patients were representative of the underlying problem population, or that the therapies were applied adequately. However, in addition to prospective experimentation, a number of other methodological protections need to be built into the test so as to guarantee that only the treatment in question and not some other factor determines the outcomes of the experiment.

Random Selection

In addition to its clinical value, a therapy's social value depends upon its ability to treat an important social problem. Therefore, the research must assure that its subjects adequately represent the underlying problem population if its findings are to be socially relevant. A study can best achieve representativeness by first identifying people suffering from the condition and then randomly selecting an appropriate number for study. Random selection prevents subtle selection biases from distorting the research sample. Nevertheless, subjects for psychotherapy outcome research are rarely selected randomly from the problem pool.

More frequently, research subjects are drawn from the pool of people who have already presented themselves for treatment, either current patients or those who apply for therapy. While this is far more convenient and inexpensive for the researcher than conducting some form of community disease survey in order to identify the true disease population, it may produce a group of subjects who are more amenable to treatment than the people with the problem who do not seek treatment. In this event, the research may only be relevant to patients who have already recognized their problems. In general, the epidemiology of most mental health conditions is not known, which presents an additional impediment to assess whether nonrandomly selected research subjects are representative of the underlying problem conditions.

Selection bias generally (either patients' self-selection for a study or the frequently imperceptible researcher biases that produce unrepresentative subject groups) is a bigger problem for psychotherapy research than for medical research that is more, although not entirely, independent of the patient's self-awareness and motivation. The frequent key to successful psychotherapy, according to many psychotherapeutic theories, is the patient's own motivation to change his or her behavior. Therefore, a research procedure biased toward the more highly motivated patient, that is, the patient who seeks treatment and who apparently already desires to change, will probably produce results that are not generally applicable to the pool of problem patients. Indeed, highly motivated patients may have already solved their problems and by pursuing therapy they may merely be searching for a ceremony to affirm their cure. Findings from this kind of biased study will most likely exaggerate the benefits of the experimental interventions.

Controls and Random Assignment

Controls assure that the outcomes are not related simply to the maturation of the subjects or to the seasonality of the disease condition. Patients frequently grow out of their problems while emotional and psychiatric problems are cyclical, alternating between periods of disease and periods of remission. Designs that simply compare patients before and after treatment cannot account for maturation and seasonality, especially in the absence of adequate epidemiological information.

Therefore, the research subjects must themselves be randomly assigned to equivalent groups; one set of groups that receive the experimental procedure, and a set of control groups that do not. The possibility of equivalence increases as the size of the sample increases. Large samples are important. The results of evaluative research are measured as the difference in outcomes between the experimental groups and the controls. Randomization assures that prior to the introduction of therapy, the control groups and the experimental groups are equivalent. In this sense nonrandomized comparison groups cannot provide assurance of comparability. Equivalence is an essential condition to assure that only the experimental condition, and not the characteristics of the research subjects themselves, accounts for the research outcomes. Crossover designs that alternately employ treatment groups as controls and controls as treatment groups even when subjects have been randomized are also susceptible to a variety of biases especially when the effects of the treatment linger.

Three types of randomized controls are possible: standard treatment controls, nontreatment controls, and placebo controls. An experimental therapy can be compared with some other therapy (e.g., a standard treatment), the most common comparison in the literature. However, if both appear to be successful (relative to the pretreatment condition of patients), then there is no indication of whether therapy was needed in the first place. In contrast, the failure of both is not necessarily evidence of ineffectiveness since both may have retarded a natural deterioration. This kind of comparison only indicates effectiveness relative to each other. Because the efficacy of treatment has generally not been established (the central argument of subsequent chapters), the viability of standard treatment controls is questionable.

Yet absolute effectiveness, the improvement over no treatment at all, is the critical issue. This can only be tested by withholding the experimental treatment from a group that is not treated at all. However, the control patient's awareness of being deprived of treatment, and, in contrast, the experimental patient's awareness of being selected for therapy, may themselves subtly affect the research outcomes. The control patient's sense of being deprived of therapy may exacerbate his or her clinical symptoms; as a result, nontreatment controls may artificially create experimental differences where none really exist. On the other hand selection for treatment may produce an effect that is unrelated to the therapy in question but only related to the fact of selection itself or to the environment of treatment.

Blinding

Clinical studies must therefore disguise, or blind, the status of the subject. This can only be achieved through placebo controls, treatmentlike structured activities that do not provide the substance of the therapy but provide the appearance of therapy. Therefore, the true effects of therapy must be measured as the difference between placebo controls and experimental groups. The comparison between nontreatment and placebo groups provides an estimate of the placebo effects of therapy.

Placebo effects can be considerable. Lambert, Weber, and Sykes (1993) reviewed a series of meta-analyses—sophisticated aggregations of individual outcome studies—that compared placebo controls with groups that received psychotherapy. They calculated a "standard effect size" of .42 for placebo effects and only .87 for psychotherapy itself. This translates into a 16 percent improvement over controls due to placebo effects, a considerable amount in comparison with the average 31 percent improvement that Lambert, Weber, and Sykes (1993) reported for psychotherapy itself. In short, Lambert, Weber, and Sykes (1993) acknowledged that more than half of the reported average benefits of psychotherapy may be due simply to placebo effects. They argued that a .42 effect size for placebo effects should simply be factored into future outcome studies of psychotherapy without actually employing the placebo controls themselves thus avoiding the ethical and legal impediments to withhold allegedly effective treatment.

While the Lambert, Weber, and Sykes (1993) suggestion for an artificial placebo adjustment reduces the complexity and cost of controlled research, it also undercuts the very basis for employing randomized controls. The viability of the Lambert, Weber, and Sykes (1993) suggestion rests upon the very shaky assumption that future outcome studies will precisely replicate the base of studies that produced the .42 effect size. However, an average placebo factor does not control for patient variation in an individual study. Although they may be valuable estimates, previous measures of placebo effects are simply inadequate substitutes for actual placebo controls.

Unfortunately, placebo controls are very difficult to construct; patients are frequently aware of their status in spite of efforts to mask whether they are in fact receiving therapy. Nevertheless, it is impossible to assess the true core of therapy—the rare skills and insights of the therapist that justify professional standing and the field's extraordinary prestige—without placebo controls.

Outcome Measures

In addition to large samples of randomly selected and assigned subjects, credible research also requires outcome measures that are standardized, objective, and reliable. In this regard the evaluators must be neutral. Measures of change in patient behaviors may be biased when they rely upon the patient's self-report, the assessment of the therapist who administers the therapy, data from collaterals (people who provide supposedly independent assessments of the patients' performance), or evaluators associated with the therapist, the therapeutic organization, or the school of therapy. Patients have obvious stakes in their outcomes and may well try to please their therapists who are important authority figures. Their collaterals may be similarly committed. The therapist is obviously not neutral, nor are the therapist's associates, students, employees, or fellow professionals. In particular, the therapist may transmit his or her expectancies for evaluation or for superficially adaptive behaviors to patients both verbally and nonverbally. The biases of self-reports and the assessments of therapists themselves have been routinely documented (e.g., Rosenthal and Rubin 1978; Dawes 1994).

Measurement itself, especially when conducted repeatedly throughout an investigation, may introduce subtle inducements for the patient to misrepresent his or her conditions. This is a notable problem when the patient feels some sense of loyalty toward the experiment. Patient loyalty can be purchased by free care, by the therapist's personal warmth, and by a belief that cure is conferred by the will and pleasure of the therapeutic situation. The problem is exacerbated when outcome information is solicited from the patient directly by his or her therapist, but the problem persists when the patient feels any sense of obligation to the therapy-giving organization or even to the therapeutic enterprise itself. Moreover, repeated applications of the same questions (some experiments applied a single questionnaire seven times in less than two years) may produce stereotypical, planned, or otherwise inaccurate responses.

One solution to the problems of iterated solicitations and patient self-reports—a greater number of randomly matched groups that are measured less frequently—imposes an immense additional cost on research. Objective and independent measures are obviously a preferable solution, avoiding these problems directly, as well as others that emerge from the expectancies of researchers and therapists. The reliability and validity of research is greatly enhanced when no one associated with the experiment has any opportunity to bias the measurement of outcomes.

In order to assure neutrality, the evaluators and the evaluations must be blind to the status of the patient. Audio and video taping are not adequate blinding devices since cues are probably present in the statements and behaviors of the patients that disclose their status in either control or treatment conditions. In a true commitment to objectivity, therapy research should actually turn over the task of assessment to evaluators who are completely independent of the therapeutic process and organization. While this is possible—a contract for evaluation to a group of statisticians or a research grant for an evaluation of therapy that is awarded to nontherapists—this has not been done. Rather, the common process, adopted by the National Institute of Mental Health and the National Institute on Drug Abuse as well as most philanthropic foundations, is to award research funds to therapists, those most committed to rosy outcomes, while hoping that a critical community of scholars will correct for professional enthusiasms in the published reports of the outcomes. Unfortunately, the psychotherapeutic community is itself a community of believers, not skeptics, with little tolerance for deviance and even less for heresy.

Furthermore, it is necessary to establish that treatment has actually been given to experimental subjects and withheld from controls. Many wait-list controls may seek out therapy from other sources while they are waiting for therapy. Experimental subjects may not have received prescribed treatments or may have failed to appear for treatment. Treatments need to be standardized and checked.

Follow-up measures over reasonably long periods of time (two years) are necessary to establish the enduring effects of therapy. Both censoring (the loss of data) and attrition (the loss of patients) has bedeviled many outcome studies. Neither loss can be assumed to be neutral. Lost data and missing patients frequently imply negative outcomes and circumscribe the analysis. There is a tendency for successful patients to maintain their availability. Follow-up evaluations and efforts to keep track of patients impose major additional costs on outcome research.

Other Pitfalls of Research

In short all of these conditions—randomized selection of subjects, random assignment, appropriate controls, objective measures, follow-up measures, blinding (patient, clinician, and researcher), assessment neutrality, large samples, and so forth—are necessary to prevent the contamination of the research. The most common contamination results from imperfectly matched groups, inappropriate controls, and subjective measures. However, other types of serious pitfalls, particularly in psychotherapy research impose an obligation for rigorous methodologies. Most of psychotherapy takes place in clinics and private offices; yet most of the research is conducted in the fishbowl of university-based research laboratories. Therefore, the research tends to mirror psychotherapy provided under optimal conditions and not its common field situation. In these laboratory conditions, the therapists tend to be better trained, the patients more highly screened, and of particular note, the therapy itself is more accountable, preventing many of the patient abuses that seem to be more common in the field.

While placebo effects can be handled by placebo controls, the broader problem of unique participation in research—a form of Hawthorne effect—is more problematic. Research situations create unique incentives for researchers, therapists, and the organization conducting the research, as well as other participants. The research usually involves a demonstration test of some particular technique with the likelihood of large future benefits if the technique proves to be effective. Consultantships, prestige, promotions, academic appointments, and even fame may be the consequences of a successful demonstration, especially if the tested technique addresses an important social problem. Successful careers have been built on programs that seemed to be able to reduce criminal activity, depression, family dysfunction, eating disorders, and substance abuse. Therefore, demonstrations usually produce extraordinary efforts among staff and therapists to produce positive results along with many opportunities for bias.

Moreover, demonstration effects may wear off, further indicating the need for follow-up measures. But even when they do not, there remains a question of whether the results were produced by common techniques or by the extraordinary efforts attendant on a critical demonstration. Short-term studies cannot get out from under this problem. Long-term studies that attempt to reach a point of routinization in treatment are required. This again, however, increases research costs.

In short, and as distinct from the objects of study in the hard sciences, participants in psychotherapeutic research—subjects, therapists, researchers, evaluators, and so on—are conscious and interact with the research environment. They pose a potential problem for research as they may tend to reflect the expectancies of the experimental situation instead of any actual improvement in their problems. This problem of expectancies can distort the reports and even the behaviors of all participants in the research situation, including the researcher whose desire to find an effective intervention and whose love of his own hypotheses may itself distort the presentation of the research. Even the subcommunity of researchers may reflect expectancy biases as a tendency to publish and fund positive findings and ignore disconfirming outcomes.

Both confirmation bias and expectancy bias are grave problems for the psychotherapy research community and more generally for the social sciences and the social services. Rosenthal and Rubin (1978) summarized 345 separate studies that estimated the degree to which the experimenter's own preferences, as distinct from the identified causative agents in the research itself, accounted for a study's outcomes. The expectancy effect is the "tendency for the experimenters to obtain results they expect, not simply because they have correctly anticipated nature's response but rather because they have helped to shape that response through their expectations" (Rosenthal and Rubin 1978, 377). These expectancies are imperceptibly conveyed to research subjects through body movements, eye contact, and a great number of other tacit and verbal cues. The authors concluded that "the reality of the phenomenon is beyond doubt and the mean size of the effect is clearly not trivial" (385). Indeed, the expectancy biases accounted for a 26 percent (.7 effect size) change in experimental subjects. Their effect in the area of psychophysical judgments, most closely related to psychotherapy research, was 35 percent (1.05 effect size). It is notable that Smith, Glass, and Miller (1980) made much of the fact that psychotherapy produced a 32 percent benefit for treated patients. However, if Rosenthal and Rubin (1978) are correct, then expectancy biases, especially in cases in which the experimenter or researcher could have affected outcomes, may account for virtually all of the change in treated patients that Smith, Glass, and Miller (1980) attributed to the therapy itself. This is a very grim possibility since without the expectancy effects, deterioration may have been reported with far greater frequency.

While RCPTs are a necessary corrective for many research pitfalls, they are not sufficient. They cannot correct for expectancy biases or other measurement distortions and they have no effect on decisions by a research community to ignore disconfirming experiments or to censor dissenting arguments. In addition to imposing the necessity for a greater rigor on psychotherapy research than on hard science, the particular problems of psychotherapy research also impose a more stringent obligation on the subcommunity of psychotherapy researchers to protect the independence and neutrality of the process of scientific discourse itself. Yet, the actual rigor of the body of psychotherapy research is an accumulation of the design decisions of individual researchers in conforming with the standards of the subcommunity of scholars. These standards that determine publication, funding, and other professional rewards, are assessments of the tolerances and demands of the larger society. In this sense, methodological rigor becomes a political statement.

Therefore, the methodological shortcomings of the body of psychotherapy research express a problem with the climate of research—the imperfections of its subcommunity of researchers—more than any inherent impediment in the research task itself. The damaged climate of the research, producing a large cloud of false and suspect evidence of effectiveness, measures the susceptibility of the subcommunity of scholars to the broader dictates of the culture.

Plan of the Book

The core chapters of this book critically examine the evidence of psychotherapy's effectiveness. The task for its concluding chapter is to explain psychotherapy's popularity and persistence in spite of the absence of credible proof that it is clinically effective and, contrary to Polsky (1991) and Dawes (1994) who both assume that the field exerts considerable independence, in spite of its political and organizational weaknesses.

It is not sufficient to simply summarize the outcome literature of psychotherapy. A variety of summary strategies have been tried, notably meta-analyses and box scores. But in driving toward conclusions of effectiveness, they have routinely obscured the many problems of research that invalidate the body of outcome research itself. Chapter 2 sets the stage for the analysis of individual outcome studies. It evaluates the earlier decades of research in the context of Smith, Glass, and Miller (1980) and it reviews other summary evaluations of psychotherapy's effectiveness subsequent to 1980. These summary statements constitute the face of psychotherapy, its generalized evidence of effectiveness that mirrors the field's effectiveness back to itself and to a larger audience outside of psychotherapy.

Because the summaries of psychotherapy research obscure the quality of the basic clinical outcome studies, the evaluation of the field's credibility requires a study-by-study analysis of its outcome statements. This is done for the recent period in chapters 3 and 4. So as to avoid tedious repetition, in each area of comment only a small number, usually one or two, of the best studies are reviewed. The large number of studies that repeat the flaws of those that are discussed at some length are simply referenced. Chapters 3 and 4 illuminate the problems of fact in psychotherapy and their broader consequences in the intellectual life of the nation by walking the arguments through the studies that are selected for analysis. Similar expositions could be made for each of the remainder of the field's research.

The studies contained in these chapters were identified by prominent summaries of the literature, notably Lambert, Christensen, and DeJulio (1986) and Gurman and Kniskern (1986), and by independent computer based searches of the literature (*Social Science Citation Index, Social Science Index, and Psychological Abstracts*) to identify randomized controlled studies subsequent to Smith, Glass, and Miller (1980). Some studies may have inadvertently been missed. Nonetheless, it is doubtful that these chapters ignore any major randomized controlled study of psychotherapy's outcomes after the benchmark of Smith, Glass, and Miller (1980).

The conclusions that are reached and the interpretation of those conclusion in chapters 5 and 6 stem out of the field's most credible testimonies to its effectiveness. The more common quality of psychotherapy research is far inferior. Moreover, since the better research tends to be performed in university-affiliated research centers under the careful scrutiny of perhaps the field's superior clinicians, the findings probably overstate the common quality of psychotherapy itself. As harsh as the conclusions may seem, the true nature of research in psychotherapy and the common quality of psychotherapy in the field are probably far inferior.

The nature of the field's research failures are discussed in chapter 5 relative to the outcomes of psychotherapy. The final chapter considers these failures more broadly in terms of the field's social meaning. Psychotherapy is not simply a failed professional exercise in reforming human behavior. The persistence of that failure, and the social tolerance for ineffective social services that it implies, speaks eloquently to the values of contemporary American culture itself. Its awe of psychotherapeutics is not based upon any feat of human engineering, but rather on psychotherapy as modern Aesopian fabulism, the creation of the myths that give coherence to society and personal life.

Unfortunately, that coherence may not conform with notions of fairness, excluding many from the bounty and social benefits of contemporary America. Taken in context of the alternatives for a more egalitarian and humane civic culture that it supplants, psychotherapy has emerged as a influential art form that reinforces the superstitious tendencies of the postmodern era.

Notes

1. Dryden and Feltham (1992) edited a series of complaints with psychotherapy, but only Eysenck and Kline went directly after the problem of undocumented effectiveness. The rest of their contributors enumerated faults within a loyal context of the field's general value. Eysenck, in going past even customary skepticism about the field's effectiveness, insisted that psychotherapy is routinely harmful. Substantiation for his position is provided later in this book.

   Rachman and Wilson (1980) are more attentive to methodological issues than many others. They provide a substantial criticism of the field's methodology, particularly for failing to control for the spontaneous remission of neurotic patients. Still, they conclude in this, the updated edition of Rachman (1971):

   > Since the First Edition was published, some slight progress has been made in the attempt to produce evidence to support the claims made on behalf of psychotherapy in general.... [I]t has to be admitted that the scarcity of convincing findings is a continuing embarrassment. Nevertheless, it is our view that modest evidence now supports the claim that psychotherapy is capable of

> producing some beneficial changes—but the negative results still outnumber the positive findings, and both of these are exceeded by reports that are beyond interpretation. (Rachman and Wilson 1980, 259)

Rachman has still been able to identify behavior therapy and cognitive behavior therapy as hopeful leads. His affection for behavior therapy is not surprising in light of his authorship of one of its early textbooks (Eysenck and Rachman 1965).

Other critics seem to easily accept the field's clinical power. According to Roustang, "The role of treatment is certainly considerable if it succeeds in clearing away a building that has been reduced to ruins but that remains in the sense that any other construction in its place is prohibited" (1983 118). He believes it does. Szasz's complaint is not that psychotherapy is ineffective since he concedes that it may help people, but that it is not truly a medical intervention. The misidentification of psychotherapy as if it were a physicochemical intervention creates a number of problems, particularly subtle coercion. But again, his criticisms are particularly cogent because he feels that psychotherapy is a successful coercive agent (Szasz 1978). Deutsch, in criticizing psychoanalysis for ignoring and distorting the psychology of women, also obviously assumes that psychoanalysis is an effective intervention (Deutsch 1980). This theme is pursued in subsequent chapters.

2. Pallone (1986) recognized that the clinical weakness of the field would support his contention that its principal utility was social; to identify bad examples for the society. "[W]e fulfill roles vital to the maintenance of a society in which visible, publicly identifiable deviance is a necessity" (69). Unfortunately, half of his citations for the contention of clinical weakness actually argue the reverse [Smith, Glass, and Miller (1980) and Bergin and Lambert (1978).] Moreover, he simply ignores the overwhelming proportion of the field's primary and secondary literature that claim that psychotherapy is effective.
3. For example, Holt (1994) held that "all that Grunbaum has done—*pace* Crews—is to make a strong a priori case that psychoanalytic data are thus contaminated; he has not proved that any particular set of free associations are useless as the basis of a given type of inference."

2

Psychotherapy's Face to the World: The Summary Assessments of its Effectiveness

The basic clinical studies of psychotherapy's effectiveness and the discussion of that body of research—intuitive reviews, box scores, and meta-analyses—have led to generally optimistic and frequently enthusiastic endorsements of psychotherapy's effectiveness. A few early summaries and evaluations of psychotherapy's outcomes, notably by Eysenck (1952, 1961, 1965), Rachman (1971), and Bergin (1971) raised substantial questions about the field's effectiveness. In contrast, later reviews seem to have resolved these doubts on the evidence of what they considered to be adequate research.

The pre-1980 Scientific Claims for the Effectiveness of Psychotherapy

Eysenck's review (1952) focused on twenty-four research articles—basic clinical studies—related to treating neurotics. He concluded that the reported improvement rates for groups that received "eclectic" therapies were as effective as for the nontreatment groups that he introduced as comparisons; psychoanalytic therapy was less effective than his controls, implying that patients may have been actually harmed by these techniques. His research was convincingly refuted on several grounds: his base of studies was weak and imprecise; his "controls" made for faulty comparisons; he made a number of errors in categorization and data analysis; and he did not include available controlled studies in his later (1965) review. "Within the framework of Eysenck's nonexperimental data base, there are limits to one's certainty about any conclusions" (Office of Technology Assessment 1980, 41).

Rachman (1971) reviewed twenty-three studies of the "verbal" psychotherapies, concluding that only one demonstrated positive outcomes. Rachman's (1971) review was also faulted, this time for his exclusion of seventeen pertinent studies.

Eysenck's work, and Rachman's as well, defined important points of skepticism, the possibility that the improvement during therapy, to the extent that it occurs, may be due to other factors such as the natural, "spontaneous" remission of the problem and placebo effects. Yet the failure of Eysenck's and Rachman's findings to withstand scrutiny did not in itself imply proof of the opposite, that psychotherapy was effective. Meltzoff and Kornreich (1970) attempted to sort through the problem of research quality by segregating methodologically credible studies that employed true controls, adequate outcome measures, and appropriate analyses from those that did not. They found that 84 percent of their credible studies yielded positive results. However, their criteria of methodological adequacy ignored a host of research considerations—measurement reactivity, blinding, expectancy biases, sample size, and so forth—that could have distorted outcomes. Meltzoff and Kornreich (1970) failed to define a core of credible research even while they may have identified patently unreliable reports.

Bergin's 1971 review of outcome studies tended to suggest that "psychotherapy, on the average, has moderate positive benefits." However, his "cross-section" of the existing literature upon which he based his conclusions contained weak, uncontrolled studies. Yet his review essay, published during a period of general social questioning, seemed to support Eysenck's charge that natural cure rates and patient deterioration may have "tempered" the effectiveness of psychotherapy. These doubts were resolved in updates of Bergin's review (Bergin and Lambert 1978; Lambert, Christensen, and DeJulio 1984; Lambert and Bergin 1994) that speciously constructed arguments for effectiveness on evidence that actually showed that psychotherapy was not much more effective than placebo controls. The following passage is cited from the "Summary and Implications" of the Bergin and Lambert (1978) essay:

> In contrast to the chapter on this topic in the previous edition of the *Handbook* (1971), wherein it was concluded that psychotherapy had an average effect that was modestly positive, recent outcome data look more favorable. A growing number of controlled outcome studies are analyzing a wide variety of therapies. These findings generally yield clearly positive results when compared with no-treatment,

> wait-list, and placebo or pseudotherapies. This may be the result of improvements in designs, but we believe that a major contributor to these newer findings is that more experienced and competent therapists have been used in recent studies. Our review of the empirical assessment of the broad range of verbal psychotherapies leads us to conclude that these methods are worthwhile when practiced by wise and stable therapists.
>
> Clearly, some people profit considerably from their therapy experience but it is disappointing to find that too often persons are not helped or are even hurt by inept applications of the very treatments that are intended to benefit them.
>
> Interpersonal and nonspecific or nontechnical factors still loom large as stimulators of patient improvements. It should come as no surprise that helping people to deal with inner conflicts, to form viable relationships, to become less threatened and defensive, or to engage in more productive behaviors can be greatly facilitated in an interpersonal relationship that is characterized by trust, warmth, acceptance, and human wisdom.
>
> These considerations imply that psychotherapy is laden with nonspecific or placebo factors...but these influences, when specified, may prove to be the essence of what provides therapeutic benefit. Instead of "controlling" for them in research designs by adopting a spurious parallel with medical placebos, we may be dismissing the active ingredients we are looking for." (179-180)

It seems more logical to conclude that these nonspecific factors argue against a psychotherapeutic approach to social problems, providing evidence that the common experiences of civilization need to be commonly provided, not that the rare skills of the therapist can compensate for their absence. Nevertheless, enthusiasm for therapy continued to grow. By 1986, Lambert, Shapiro, and Bergin concluded that credible research had convincingly refuted the skeptics. Psychotherapy was highly effective, long lasting, and related to the skill of the therapist:

> Many psychotherapies that have been subjected to empirical study have been shown to have demonstrable effects on a variety of clients. These effects are not only statistically significant but clinically meaningful. Psychotherapy facilitates the remission of symptoms. It not only speeds up the natural healing process but often provides additional coping strategies and methods for dealing with future problems. Psychologists, psychiatrists, social workers, and marriage and family therapists as well as patients can be assured that a broad range of therapies, when offered by skillful, wise, and stable therapists, are likely to result in appreciable gains for the client.

Luborsky, Singer, and Luborsky (1975), in a review of thirty-three studies, and Parloff (1978), in an exhaustive review of the literature (apparently intended for the annual budget hearings in Congress on behalf of the National Institutes of Mental Health), concluded that psychotherapy is generally successful. Gurman and Kniskern (1978b) and (1986) reached similarly positive conclusions for family therapy, estimating that "non behavioral marital and family therapies produce beneficial outcomes in about two-thirds of cases, and their effects are superior to non treatment" (Gurman and Kniskern 1986, 572).

In reviewing the body of the field's primary studies and its critical literature, Congress' Office of Technology Assessment (OTA) reached the conclusion that psychotherapy was frequently cost effective. OTA (1980) also implicitly reached the conclusion that the existing base of research was not easily amenable to cost/benefit comparisons. Nevertheless, OTA (1980) found

> good evidence of psychotherapy's positive effects. Although this evidence may not be generalizable to the wide range of problems for which therapy is employed, it suggests that additional research may provide data useful for the development of mental health policy. (5)

The Problems of the Reviews and the Benchmark of Smith, Glass, and Miller (1980)

Each of these prominent reviews of outcome studies and many far weaker reviews as well attempted to systematically evaluate the findings of the multitude of accumulated claims (literally thousands of studies) for the benefits of psychotherapy in order to reach conclusions about its general effectiveness. The tasks they faced were not simply to tabulate and to sort through the different problems, patients, therapies, and outcomes, but also to develop a meaningful weighting system that would favor methodologically rigorous and theoretically important studies. These summaries produced pivotal judgments regarding the field's effectiveness and its social value.

The review strategies for comparing and summarizing the outcomes of individual studies fell into three general types: intuitive methods, box scores, and meta-analyses. All three types commented on methodology and the prospect of bias, but usually as an afterthought in making a plea for more rigorous research. There was little appreciation for the possibility that psychotherapy's reported cures, like Uri Geller's bent spoons, were mirages created in methodological deserts. The fact that the findings of the different studies tended to converge mattered more to almost all reviewers than their individual credibility. The credibility of each study was assumed in deference to collegial courtesy that the scientific milieu of the field—psychology as a social *science*—would naturally guard rigor.

The intuitive summaries simply presented the base of primary research in an individualistic, frequently literary manner and evaluated it against stated or implicit criteria. Some of these intuitive reviews, in particular the two series by Bergin and by Gurman in the different editions of the *Handbook of Psychotherapy and Behavior Change,* were thorough and exhaustive, but still highly subjective in the way they went about weighing evidence and drawing conclusions. However, most of the intuitive summaries were neither thorough nor particularly astute; they were frank partisan salvos in the conflict among competitive psychotherapeutic camps.

The second type of summary, typified by Luborsky, Singer, and Luborsky's box-score analysis (1975), was explicit in its methods, but limited by a reliance upon crude analytic techniques that did not allow for much more than the tabulation of outcomes. The third type of analysis was objective and systematic, but unlike the box-score techniques, it permitted the researcher to disaggregate, weight, and recombine the separate findings of different studies. This latter group of techniques is generally referred to as meta-analysis with Smith, Glass, and Miller (1980) becoming a crucial point of development in both the field's methods and its evaluation of itself. Smith, Glass, and Miller (1980) and other meta-analyses continue to focus debate within the field.

Meta-analytic techniques permitted a reviewer to compare the effects of therapeutic interventions across studies. This statistical process produced a standardized measure of the impact of the treatment—its "effect size"—that indicated, depending upon the measure, the percentage of patients who benefited from therapy and the degree of their change.

Effect sizes could be calculated for a single study or for a variety of studies. Studies could be grouped by any of their characteristics and quantitative statements could be made about their effectiveness, that is, their average effect size. Effect sizes were amenable to further quantitative analyses—a variety of regression techniques—against any of their characteristics that could be quantified, including "dummy" variables of nominal qualities (e.g., client diagnosis, gender, form of publication). Unfortunately, many of these characteristics (e.g., the quality of a study's methods) are not easily translated into meaningful continuous measures.

Smith, Glass, and Miller (1980) identified 475 reliable, controlled outcomes studies that they felt adhered to "the acknowledged canons of experimental science" (8).

> All controlled studies of the effectiveness of any form of psychotherapy formed the population of interest for this project.... No form of psychotherapy was excluded if the therapy (1) involved clients identified by themselves or others; (2) if the clients sought or were referred for treatment; (3) if the treatment or intervention was psychological or behavioral; and (4) if the person delivering the treatment was identified as a psychotherapist by virtue of training or professional interest. (Smith, Glass, and Miller 1980, 55–56)

Studies were compared across eighteen considerations: the date of the study and its form of publication; the experimenter's professional affiliation, allegiance, and experience; the degree of blinding; the client's diagnosis, similarity to the therapist, and intelligence; whether clients were analogues or real patients; the process of assignment to research groups (i.e., randomization); attrition; internal validity; the type and duration of the therapy; the modality; and the type and reactivity of the outcome measures.

Smith, Glass, and Miller (1980) found that psychotherapy was basically effective. "[T]he average person who would score at the 50th percentile of the untreated control population, could expect to rise to the 80th percentile with respect to that population after receiving psychotherapy." In addition,

> little evidence was found for the alleged existence of negative effects of psychotherapy.... Only 9 percent of the effect sizes were negative.... Nor was there convincing evidence in the dispersion on the treated groups that some members became better and some worse as a result of psychotherapy. (88)

Some of the therapies, cognitive therapies in particular, appeared to be very effective. Patients given some form of the cognitive therapies would be better off than 99 percent of the control groups after therapy. Yet, other interventions such as "reality therapy" produced only small but still positive results.

When possible, Smith, Glass, and Miller (1980) compared the published outcomes of therapy to groups that had received no treatment at all (wait-list controls) and to controls that had received placebo treatment (usually time structured, nontherapeutic activities given in a group). Smith, Glass, and Miller (1980) argued that experimental group outcomes could appropriately be compared with nontreatment controls, that placebo controls were not necessary. Indeed, Bergin and Lambert's (1978) later conversion to belief in the general effectiveness of psychotherapy stemmed out of their contention that the placebo effect was actually an essential therapeutic ingredient of successful treatment. Smith, Glass, and Miller's (1980) large positive results from comparisons with nontreated controls that were not placebos shrank greatly in comparison with placebo treatments. Only cognitive treatment was more than 10 percent superior to placebos.

Their correlational analysis supported their theme, although with a few provocative findings. The reactivity of measurement showed the largest (although still small) correlation with effect size. In other words, the degree to which measures were susceptible to the biases of the researchers and other evaluators of outcomes accounted for a portion of the effect sizes. Moreover, when patients were evaluated at follow-up points after treatment, their therapeutic gains fell as much as 50 percent. The duration of the therapy itself did not seem to be associated with its benefits.

> The characteristics of a therapy... bore surprisingly little relation to the size of effect. Individual therapy and group therapy and combinations of them were equally effective... (however) the characteristics of the clients involved in the therapy evaluation influenced the size of the effects eventually produced. Depressed clients and clients with simple, monosymptomatic phobias were associated with the largest effects; psychotics, neurotics, and handicapped clients with the smallest. (125)

By the mid-1980s and continuing today, methodological adequacy for research in psychotherapy has been largely satisfied by randomized controls, quantitative measures, and quantitative analyses. However, these necessary characteristics of credible research are insufficient by themselves to protect against fundamental threats to credibility. There has been little sensitivity to the possibility that evidence for efficacy may have been growing proportionate to the fields needs, cutting the cloth of proof to fit a body of ambitions. Reasonable skepticism, certainly tenable in light of the widespread sociological truism that defined growth at any price as an organizational imperative, pointed to the possibility that the field's desires were realized in *reports* of client benefits, perhaps through the expectancies of researchers and practitioners, without being expressed in meaningful behavior changes among patients.

In spite of their many scientific transgressions, the vast majority of the outcome reviews of psychotherapy, notably Smith, Glass, and Miller

(1980) and even those that rely upon intuitive methods, reiterated the field's basic commitment to scientific methods. Most of them agree on the form of optimal research even while they differ over the compromises with rigor that still maintain scientific credibility.

Smith, Glass, and Miller (1980) and the Later Reviews of Studies

The summaries, the studies of studies, repeat the distortions of the base of primary outcome research, carrying through their near-uniform enthusiasm for the value of psychotherapy. These reviews are important ideological statements. They package the collective judgments of the field, a sense of its social value, for public policy and social approval. They are the field's attempts to speak broadly to its constituency.

Yet, the basic requirement—adequate research methodologies—for reaching any judgment that is scientifically credible on the effectiveness of treatment is missing. The claims for effectiveness themselves provide an estimate of the problem. The meta-analyses have come up with only small estimates of the superiority of psychotherapy over any controls. Indeed, a reanalysis of Smith, Glass, and Miller (1980) defines a Wild West of therapeutic outcomes and the persistent likelihood, reflecting the tyranny of grouped data, that many patients deteriorate during the course of therapy. Moreover, even its slight meta-analytic edge is lost in the background static of the consistent pitfalls of psychotherapy research and the expectancy biases of its researchers and practitioners.

For much of the field, the issue of its effectiveness has been settled by the more prominent of these reviews, in particular Smith, Glass, and Miller (1980), that provided the field with a comprehensive meta-analytic benchmark of its outcomes. Yet their procedures and even their data cannot support their optimism.

First, Smith, Glass, and Miller (1980) handled their comparison with placebos in a self-serving manner, preferring comparisons with nontreatment groups. However, following the logic of rigorous clinical science, the true effect of an intervention, its true effect size, is measured by the benefits it confers above a placebo. The fact that their reported placebo effects are so large in comparison with their treatment effects [effects sizes of .56 (21.2 percent) versus .86 (30.5 percent)] suggests that the added effect of psychotherapy above nonprofessional time-structured activities is very small, on the order of 10 percent. Yet, even this small increment is doubtful in light of their own evidence that measurement reactivity accounted for more than 3 percent of the effect size variance.

Second, and contrary to their initial claims that they only included rigorous studies, the Smith, Glass, and Miller (1980) meta-analysis contained both analogue studies, studies that were not controlled, and more importantly, studies whose outcomes did not reach statistical significance (in other words, differences that could be due to chance itself). They actually contradicted their avowed commitment to science by condemning rigorous standards as a "devise for cutting" the outcome literature. They criticized previous reviews, especially those that questioned the efficacy of psychotherapy for arbitrarily imposing

> "textbook" standards; these methodological rules, learned as dicta in graduate school and regarded as the touchstone of publishable articles in prestigious journals, were applied arbitrarily; for example, note again Rachman's high-handed dismissal on methodological grounds of study after study of psychotherapy outcome. (38)

Third, the issue of patient deterioration in psychotherapy is persistent. The frequent rejections of the possibility of patient deterioration (May 1971; Mays and Franks 1980; Bergin and Lambert 1978; Lambert, Shapiro, and Bergin 1986) occupy a curious position, hiding behind the methodological weaknesses of the field by insisting that the burden to prove harm is on the shoulders of the critic and not on the shoulders of the therapist. They argued that because the research fails to *credibly* demonstrate harm, the charge of deterioration is still indeterminate and probably false. However, they fail to extend their argument to the observation that the outcome literature fails also to credibly test *any* effect of psychotherapy, not just its deterioration effects. In contrast, Smith, Glass, and Miller (1980), in a long discussion of the obligations of research, set the burden of proof firmly on the shoulders of the interventionist.

While the Smith, Glass, and Miller (1980) data seem to refute the challenge of deterioration, a reanalysis of their data support it. These recomputations imply that a huge proportion of the effect sizes of a normal distribution of effect sizes would fall below the "0" score, that is, the score for nontreatment. For example, 8 percent of the effect sizes for psychodynamic therapy would fall below "0"; 36 percent for reality therapy; 14 percent for behavior therapy; and 27 percent for systematic desensitization (Epstein 1984a). The amount of estimated deterioration increases beyond even these points proportionate to the extent to which reported outcomes exaggerate positive effects.

Throughout their analysis, Smith, Glass, and Miller (1980) presented effect sizes of the different therapies as though they were populations of outcomes instead of samples drawn from the underlying populations. Following the more tenable assumption that the grouped effect sizes are actually a distribution of sample means and not individual cases, the underlying distributions of the population of effect sizes and their standard deviations increase dramatically. Their assumed standard deviations are really standard errors. Even assuming modest sample sizes of twenty-five, variations become so large that in many cases almost 50 percent of patient outcomes fall below zero effect size, that is, into the area of negative effects relative to nontreatment controls (Epstein 1984a).[1]

These huge variations suggest that the benefits of psychotherapy are wildly unpredictable. Yet, these data may underestimate the actual amount of deterioration since the recomputations make no adjustment for placebo effects, reactivity, expectancy biases, and misreporting.

Furthermore, many of the studies were conducted under optimal conditions of therapy, by highly regarded and responsible therapists in research situations. For all their problems and uncertain outcomes, they may yet be best-case estimates of the reality of psychotherapy as it is commonly practiced. The actual conditions of psychotherapy for the typical patient may be a far more uncaring, abusive, and unprofessional experience.

Finally, Smith and Glass (1977), in their early version of the Smith, Glass, and Miller (1980) study, commented on the curiosity that the benefit rate for psychotherapy measured by their analysis was almost the same as measured by Eysenck in his earlier "tendentious diatribes in which he claimed to prove that 75 percent of neurotics got better regardless of whether or not they were in therapy" (Smith and Glass 1977, 752). Since Smith and Glass (1977) did not explicitly adjust for the "seasonality" of the different conditions that were being treated, their study would seem to corroborate Eysenck's skepticism if not actually his work.

Subsequent to Smith, Glass, and Miller (1980), summaries of outcome studies—intuitive discussions, box scores, and meta-analyses—have usually been even more encouraging in pointing to the benefits of separate treatments and treatment conditions. On the basis of a meta-analysis of 163 treatment/control comparisons of psychotherapy outcomes for children, Weisz et al. (1987) found that treated groups averaged an effect size of .79, ending up 29 percent better off than controls. Casey and Berman (1985) had reported an effect size of .71 for children in therapy, implying that treated children were 26 percent better off than controls. Howard, Kopta, and Krause (1986), in applying probit analysis to "15 diverse sets of data from their own research and from research previously reported in the literature" over the past thirty years, concluded that the relationship between length of psychotherapeutic treatment and patient benefit was such that "by 8 sessions approximately 50 percent of patients are measurably improved, and approximately 75 percent are improved by 26 sessions" (159). Patterson (1984) found that even Bergin's reviews were too cautious and biased:

> Considering the obstacles to research on the relationship between therapist variables and therapy outcomes, the magnitude of the evidence is nothing short of amazing. There are few things in the field of psychology for which the evidence is so strong. The evidence for the necessity, if not the sufficiency, of the therapist conditions of accurate empathy, respect, or warmth, and therapeutic genuineness is incontrovertible. (437)

Miller and Berman (1983) concluded on the basis of forty-eight studies that "cognitive behavior therapies were superior to no treatment; however there was no firm evidence that these therapies were superior to other psychotherapies" (39). Tillitski (1990) compared the effectiveness of different psychotherapeutic approaches. In the same manner, a variety of different summaries of outcome studies found consistent grounds for the effectiveness of psychotherapy of one form or another in the treatment of fear (Glaister 1982), headache (Blanchard and Andrasik 1982; Blanchard et al. 1980), insomnia (Borkovec 1982), bulimia (Fettes and Peters 1992), and anorexia nervosa (Hsu 1980) and others.

The basic Smith, Glass, and Miller (1980) meta-analysis has been corroborated and extended by a number of studies (Landman and Dawes 1982; Shapiro 1985). The Andrews and Harvey (1981) meta-analysis concluded that psychotherapy was highly effective with neurotic patients. Shapiro and Shapiro's (1982b) meta-analysis produced the finding that "consistent with previous reviews, the mean of the 1,828 effect size measures obtained from the 414 treated groups approached one standard deviation unit, and differences among treatment methods accounted for, at most, 10 percent of the variance in effect size" (581). Giblin, Sprenkle, and Sheehan's (1985) meta-analysis of premarital, marital, and family interventions produced an average effect size of .44, "which indicated that the average person who participated in enrichment is better off following intervention than 67 percent of those who do not." (257)

Steinbrueck, Maxwell, and Howard (1983) conducted a meta-analysis of fifty-six outcome studies of the relative effectiveness of psychotherapy and drug therapy in the treatment of unipolar depression and concluded that psychotherapy was more effective than drug therapy. The Dush, Hirt, and Schroeder (1983) meta-analysis

> resulted in the conclusion that self-statement modification psychotherapy maintained an advantage beyond typical placebo effects of at least two-thirds of its advantage over no-treatment. These effects were durable over time and apparently independent of the observed methodological flaws of the studies. Spontaneous recovery, coincidental change, and atheoretical therapy benefits fell well short of the change fostered by self-statement modification.... Self-statement modifications's average level of effectiveness lends it favorable status among alternative psychotherapies. (418)

But the interpretative summaries, meta-analytic and others, are not credible. Their base of primary research does not contain even one credible test of outcomes. The buoyant optimism of most of these summaries have overwhelmed the field's few critical voices that call attention to the inherent weakness of the research (e.g., Strube and Harmann 1982; Shapiro and Shapiro 1982a; Prioleau, Murdock, and Brody 1983).

The clear but infrequent voice of the critical tradition in psychotherapy has been largely ignored. One of the rare notes of skepticism that reached into the empirical data itself, Prioleau, Murdock, and Brody (1983) reanalyzed the most credible portion of the Smith, Glass, and Miller (1980) data set, the thirty-two studies in which psychotherapy was compared with a *placebo control.* They found that the median effect size was only .15, representing an improvement over placebo control of only 6 percent; the mean placebo effect size was .42 which is still only a 16 percent improvement. Both were considerably less than the Smith, Glass, and Miller (1980) reported mean effect size of .85 (30 percent improvement) for all studies with *any control.* Yet even these thirty-two studies, presumably the cream of the crop, are so lax in protecting against researcher and therapist biases, that the possibility cannot be ignored that psychotherapy may actually be consistently harmful. The fact that the field has flourished in spite of Prioleau, Murdock, and Brody (1983) strongly suggests that the meaning of psychotherapy does not lie in its explicit function as a rational method for curing, preventing, or rehabilitating those who suffer from mental health problems.

The Summary Reviews of Family Psychotherapy

The summary reviews of family psychotherapy outcome studies, when they uncritically accepted the base of studies, were positive. The meta-analytic approach was employed by many of the more recent reviews so as to avoid the "inherent subjectivity" of more narrative approaches (Hahlweg and Markman 1988, 440). In the ten years or so prior to the early 1980s—that is, the period of time just before the acceptance of meta-analytic techniques as the state of the art for summarizing a group of outcome studies—many review judgments were positive even while they were qualified as emergent, promising, or hopeful because of the methodologically "diverse" sources of data for their conclusions.

"Family therapy for drug abuse is gaining widespread acceptance and shows considerable promise for dealing effectively with problems of this type" (Stanton 1979, 251). "Although the superiority of conjoint family therapy has not been established over nonconjoint methods, both are superior to no treatment at all" (DeWitt 1978). Gurman found that "the overall improvement rate (for marital enrichment programs) across a heterogeneous collection of patients, therapists, and treatment modalities was 66 percent, suggesting, conservatively at least, a moderately positive therapeutic effect in light of the judgment that 'spontaneous' rates appear to be much lower in marital than in individual therapy" (Gurman 1973, 145). However, a few years later in reviewing similar outcome studies (marital as well as premarital enrichment programs), Gurman and Kniskern found several deficiencies in the base of studies that comprised the source for this conclusion that "require a cautious optimism about the efficacy" of family therapy (Gurman and Kniskern 1977, 3).

One year later, these authors fiercely criticized the methodological shortcomings of the marital therapy research:

> Our purpose has been to keep behavioral couples therapy in a broader empirical perspective. As active marital therapists and marital therapy researchers, we are not overwhelmed by the quality of objective study in the marital and family therapy field. While we have our own theoretical and clinical biases and beliefs that incor-

> porate, but do not emphasize, behavioral thinking, we encourage, even dogmatically expect, marital and family therapists of all theoretical persuasions to remain "open to the data," from wherever they derive and whatever they may show. (Gurman and Kniskern 1978, 146)

After taking to task a number of reviews of behavioral marital therapy for deriving conclusions on the basis of flawed research, Gurman and Kniskern (1978) then go on to cite methodologically weaker studies—ten analogue studies and thirteen studies of naturalistic couples—that question the value of behavioral marital therapy. Nevertheless, Olson, Russell, and Sprenkle (1980), as well as Beck (1975) concluded that marital therapy generally had gained credibility and had emerged as a viable treatment approach for most mental health problems. In a similar way, Wells and Dezen (1978) reviewed studies of nonbehavioral family therapies that appeared between 1971 and 1976. They identified twenty studies that met their minimal criteria for methodological rigor—random assignment, measurements before and after treatment, and an appropriate statistical analysis. They concluded that "family therapy has not been able to demonstrate more than equivalence with nonformal treatment," that is, a nontreatment control (267). Nevertheless, they still insisted that

> at a very broad level it is apparent that family therapy—in the nonbehavioral form reviewed—has been legitimized. As a means of delivering helping services, family therapy can no longer be viewed as a rank newcomer of uncertain validity and doubtful status. Both the methodologically adequate studies and certain of the studies judged to be methodologically inadequate contribute to this general legitimizing effect. (267)

Jacobson et al.'s (1984) reanalysis of outcome data reaffirmed the value of behavioral marital therapy, although with cautious reference to methodological problems. "Slightly more than half of the couples improved...deterioration was rare...the majority of couples maintained whatever gains they had made" (497). Wampler's (1982a) summary of nineteen separate studies "indicates that [the couples communication program] is an effective program in teaching communication skills to couples. The evidence is particularly strong when behavioral measures of couple interaction were used" (351). Sprenkle and Storm (1983) supported the efficacy of divorce therapy:

> There is strong evidence for the superiority of mediation to traditional adversary methods.... Conciliation counseling appears to increase the number of reconciliations in the short-term. (239)

Meta-analysis did not reduce the positive tenor of earlier conclusions. Giblin, Sprenkel, and Sheehan (1985) "lay to rest the charge that 'enrichment is ineffective.'" Their base of eighty-five controlled studies included all programs that provided some form of marital enrichment treatment, not just behavioral therapy. While their analysis defined an effect size of .44, twice that of Hahlweg and Markman (1988) (see below), they concluded that it "indicates that the average person who participates in enrichment is better off following intervention than 67 percent of those who do not" (269). However, the positive effects were not sustained over time. It is noteworthy that they found that larger effect sizes were more often associated with behavioral measures stemming from videotaping or audiotaping than with the self-report measures of patients. While the authors assume that many behavioral measures are more objective, they ignore the possibility that they may also be subject to the expectancy biases of researchers.

Moreover, the patient behaviors that are assumed to indicate therapeutic outcome may not be valid indicators of true remission, or may merely be a temporary adaptation to the research situation. In this light, the disjuncture between what clients report and what researchers report is very suggestive, especially since gains in the Giblin, Sprenkle, and Sheehan (1985) meta-analysis were not generally sustained at follow-up.

Hahlweg and Markman's (1988) meta-analysis reached similarly positive conclusions, finding large and stable benefits for both behavioral marital therapy and premarital intervention—effect sizes of .95 (32.9 percent) and .79 (28.5 percent), respectively—that were stable over time. Their meta-analysis reviewed twenty-four studies that employed some form of control group. "The average rate of improvement after therapy that is attributable to behavior marital therapy is about 40 percent" (445). They are generally complimentary about the quality of the studies that they review.

However, in the few cases when the reviewer went beyond the requirement of a control group to raise more thoroughgoing methodological issues, the value of family therapy became much more uncertain. Bagarozzi and Rauen (1981) were able to identify only thirteen studies of premarital counseling programs that met their very minimal criteria for methodological rigor—standardized intervention procedures and outcome measures to assess effectiveness. They concluded that

> although premarital counseling programs are on the rise in the United States, no empirical data exist to support the notion that these programs reduce the inci-

> dence of divorce or separation for those couples who participate, because the follow-up evaluations which have been conducted thus far have not allowed sufficient time to elapse after treatment to obtain a valid measure of their effectiveness. Similarly, no data exist which indicate that couples who participate in premarital counseling programs are more satisfied or successful in their marriages than those who do not. Finally, we do not know whether premarital counseling practices serve any prophylactic functions; for example, do they prevent bad marriages from taking place. (27)

Masten (1979) concluded that "if the value of family therapy as a treatment alternative or, ideally, as the 'treatment of choice' for a referred individual child is to be established, more and better controlled comparative outcome studies will be necessary."

Constructing the Face of Psychotherapy

The clinical value of psychotherapy hinges on the quality of the studies that describe its benefits. The many summaries that uncritically accepted this base of research naturally reach a conclusion of reassuring effectiveness—that the short-term, inexpensive, and socially compatible interventions of psychotherapy can prevail against embedded personal problems. Yet, a long list of methodological pitfalls subvert Smith, Glass, and Miller's (1980) happy conclusions and raise doubts about the rest of the field's many corroborating summary statements: small samples, the absence of blinding and appropriate controls, researcher biases (including the likelihood of expectancy biases), nonrepresentative samples, poor descriptions of interventions, short study periods, and so forth. A prudent skepticism has been ignored both in the research and in the critical literature of its community of social scientists. The climate in which the field conducts its research is inimical to objective, unbiased science. Rigorous methodological precautions are not in place to guard the integrity of findings against social preferences and the lure of government funding, the personal stakes of the researchers and the therapists, the stakes of their host research organizations—usually universities—and the frequent privateering interests of entrepreneurs.

The psychotherapy research covering the outcomes of individual, group, and family treatments since the publication of Smith, Glass, and Miller (1980)—the subjects for the next two chapters—repeats the failures of earlier studies. In spite of some improvement over the past few decades in the use of randomization, quantification, and multiple objective outcome measures, the methodologies are still too porous to sustain any conclusion except that the outcomes of individual and group psychotherapy are indeterminate at best, probably ineffective, and possibly harmful. Without a demonstrable clinical value, the ideological uses of psychotherapy in contemporary social and political discourse stands out as the field's principal function and the reason for its persistence.

Note

1. In retabulating Smith, Glass, and Miller's (1980) reported effect sizes, "instead of assuming that each therapy group of effect sizes is a population of outcomes...the more tenable assumption should be made that they represent a sample of findings out of a population of effect sizes. Following this assumption, certain characteristics about this underlying population of effect sizes emerge that are very damaging to claims that psychotherapy produces consistently beneficial effects" (Epstein 1984a, 167). If the assumption is made that the samples of the studies that produced the effect sizes contained either twenty-five subjects each or 100 subjects each, then the reported standard deviations should be adjusted in the following way for selected therapies (the complete retabulations are found in Epstein 1984a, 168, table 3):

Therapy	**Mean ES**[1]	**SD**[2]	**n=25**[3]	**n=100**[4]
Psychodynamic	0.69	0.50	2.5	5.0
Hypnotherapy	1.82	1.15	5.8	11.5
Cognitive-behavioral	1.13	0.83	4.2	8.3
Systematic desensitization	1.05	1.58	7.9	15.8
Placebo treatment	0.56	1.25	6.3	12.5

[1] Mean effect sizes as reported by Smith, Glass, and Miller (1980)
[2] Standard deviations for each mean effect size as reported by Smith, Glass, and Miller (1980)
[3] Recomputed standard deviation assuming a sample size of 25
[4] Recomputed standard deviation assuming a sample size of 100

As examples, assuming n=25, 39 percent of psychodynamic patients and 40 percent of cognitive-behavioral patients are worse off than nontreatment controls. Even if the effect sizes of reported treatments are not discounted by the placebo effect to define a true zero effect score, the percent falling in the area of negative effects is still substantial in each case, approaching 50 percent. Adjustments for placebo effects and for greater sample sizes increase even these large estimates of harm.

3

Recent Tests of the Effectiveness of Individual and Group Psychotherapy

The summary assessments of psychotherapy are only as accurate as their base of primary studies. In turn, those outcome studies of psychotherapy are conducted with the precise purpose of evaluating the social and clinical utility of specific interventions. Outcome studies are the quality assurance tests for establishing effectiveness. They also measure the insight and rigor of the community of psychotherapists and psychotherapy scholars.

At least formally, the psychotherapeutic community has accepted the process of science as a bulwark against becoming a grab bag of bogus cures, a resurrected spiritualism for the twentieth-century soul. As a consequence, the virtue of objective, coherent, and controlled testing is adopted in order to establish the viability of psychotherapeutic treatments. These tests create strategic properties that the psychotherapeutic community exhibits to prove that treatment can successfully modify dysfunctional behaviors and to promote psychotherapy as a tool of social policy.

The outcome studies that are analyzed in these chapters provide the most rigorous and theoretically sophisticated recent evidence for psychotherapy's effectiveness. They were published in prestigious refereed journals between 1980, when Smith, Glass, and Miller was published, through 1992 and cited in prominent summary reviews of psychotherapy (such as Lambert, Shapiro, and Bergin 1986).[1] These studies attempt to settle important issues of practice and theory while they employ randomized designs and other features of superior research. Uncontrolled studies, studies with historical controls, and otherwise methodologically weak studies are ignored. In this way, the studies that are discussed are the most scientific tests and, therefore, the most credible statements of the effectiveness of psychotherapy since 1980. The common quality of the contemporary psychotherapy research, while representing a general improvement over the quality of research in the field prior to Smith, Glass, and Miller (1980), falls off steeply from these studies, imperfect as they are. As a result, the criticism of this pool of superior research understates the actual deficiencies of the field's tests of its effectiveness.

A number of major sources—especially the American Psychiatric Association's *Treatments of Psychiatric Disorders* (hereafter referred to as TPD 1989)—provide reference points for psychotherapeutic theory and treatment. The TPD is an immense compendium produced by a task force of the American Psychiatric Association; it is a definitive statement of current practice. At a minimum, it represents the range of treatments that carry the cachet of perhaps the principal psychotherapeutic organization in the United States today.

However, the TPD—as well as many other psychotherapy texts—share a common and serious failure. They tend to divorce their prescriptions for treatment from the credibility of the studies that establish their basic authority. Notwithstanding a variety of weak disclaimers and qualifications, these works subtly provide a reassuring but misleading rationality in recommending a variety of treatments. Locutions such as "it appears that," "it could be concluded," and "the literature tends to suggest" fail to discount the actual findings of the outcome studies by the pitfalls of their methods. Thus, the enthusiasm of the field for its alphabetized and indexed practice wisdom prevails over scientific caution.

The following analyses correct this failure by closely tying the actual outcomes of the research to its methodology. The result is to question the field's professional authority, resting as it does upon very flawed information.

The pool of recent outcome research focused either on specific disorders or on specific treatments. The studies tested the effectiveness of psychotherapy in treating the range of personal disorders and complaints that underpin many social problems: neurosis, sexual abuse, headache, insomnia, hypertension, anxiety in children, posttraumatic stress disorder, depression, chronic pain, anorexia nervosa, panic disorder, agoraphobia, attention deficit disorder, and drug and alcohol addiction. The outcome studies also compared the effectiveness of different treatments:

brief therapy, flooding and implosive therapy, culturally sensitive psychotherapy, assertion training, cognitive therapy, hypnosis, behavior therapy, cognitive-behavior therapy, systematic desensitization, dynamic group psychotherapy, and others.

The Social and Theoretical Value of Psychotherapy

The social value of contemporary psychotherapy rests on its promise to correct dysfunctional behavior in a short amount of time and with little cost. The typical course of therapy in the contemporary literature was administered in relatively few sessions, frequently no more than fifteen weekly meetings that usually lasted no more than 90 minutes. Clearly, demonstrations of effectiveness tend to validate the type of therapy that was employed; however, they also tend to support the theoretical underpinnings of the therapy—the assumptions about the nature of dysfunctional behavior and the interventions that are required to change those behaviors.

A fierce debate—notably in the treatment of depression—has been waged between the variety of psychotherapeutic schools over the effectiveness and, consequently, the social value of their different theoretical approaches. To the extent to which any approach is successful, the core of its therapeutic interchange constitutes valuable wisdom, the knowledge of how to reduce personal problems. Scientific tests of effectiveness separate true wisdom from bogus cure.

General Characteristics of the Contemporary Pool of Outcome Studies

The best studies in the contemporary pool of outcome research tested short-term interventions. Sample sizes were typically small. Samples in few studies exceeded fifty. Many samples contained fewer than fifteen subjects. The largest sample for a clinical study contained only eighty-four patients. Many studies employed legitimate patients who were recruited from active treatment or live waiting lists. Some advertised for patients and in other ways employed analogues for real patients or produced groups of atypical patients through selective sampling procedures. Small samples open the door to expectancy biases and reduce the ability of the study to detect slight outcomes. Atypical samples severely circumscribe the applicability of the results to the larger populations of need.

The therapists themselves who performed the treatments and the settings of therapy may not have been representative of psychotherapeutic practice. Most studies were conducted in university-affiliated research centers while the therapists were usually professors and researchers or their students. Very few of the studies employed therapists outside of the research center itself or in any way drew their samples of therapists so as to represent the therapeutic conditions of live practice. In the end, the therapies were probably provided by superior clinicians working in optimal settings. As a consequence, the reported outcomes of therapy are probably exaggerated estimates of the more customary patient experience.

Research Methods

Many studies randomized subjects to a standard treatment control and less frequently either to a nontreatment control or to a placebo control. Others, the common coin of the journals but ignored in this review, still employed case study procedures and used subjects as their own controls in "quasi-experimental" designs. Although random assignment seems to be far more common in the very recent cohort of studies than in studies prior to Smith, Glass, and Miller (1980), it is still not a hallmark of outcome research, nor even a requirement for publication in the field's leading journals.

Moreover, nontreatment controls, especially placebos, are still not widely employed since the effectiveness of psychotherapy seems to be a settled issue that affects research design. "[W]e chose to dispense with no-treatment controls, in view of our specific interest in comparing treatments, the ethical and logistical difficulties attending the use of such controls and the overall evidence for the efficacy of psychotherapies" (Shapiro et al. 1990, 99). The most common control group is still a standard treatment control, that is, some other form of therapy. Not surprisingly, the most common finding is that the experimental treatment is as effective as the standard treatment control, echoing the Luborsky, Singer, and Luborsky (1975) conclusion that everyone wins. However, without a rigorous substantiation of the effectiveness of the standard treatment, the more logical conclusion would seem to be that all outcomes are indeterminate.

Measures

Studies frequently employed standardized interviewer assessments (e.g., the Beck Depression Inventory and the Hamilton Rating Scale for Depression) in combination with other kinds of structured patient reports. In pursuit of more objective and reliable measurement of outcome behaviors, some studies audio- and videotaped client behaviors during the therapy sessions, then submitted those tapes to supposedly neutral judges. Infrequently, tapes were rated by judges who were neither the therapist nor the researcher; however, even this level of independence was often not maintained.

Studies employed a wide variety of outcome measures and instruments to collect data, although some studies relied upon only a few measures. The reported inter-rater reliability scores of the measures ranged widely from rare high Kappas of over .95 to more common scores well under .75. It is likely that even the modest reported reliabilities were inflated by irregularities in the testing procedures and that the instruments themselves as applied to the live research situation tolerated a substantial amount of differential bias. The imperfect reliabilities of the scales and instruments seem to pose more than a hurdle for the research itself. The imperfections of the instruments and the suspect conditions under which their psychometric properties were defined appear to open the door to the possibility of many reporting biases and not simply to a great amount of random noise. Unreliable measures would mask true differences between the experimental and control groups, but biased measures would exaggerate the differences.[2]

Moreover, raters were frequently graduate and undergraduate students, usually in psychology or psychiatry, some of whom performed their tasks for course credit and some of whom were paid. At follow-up, the ratings usually relied upon patient self-reports and rarely upon direct behavioral observations. Follow-up interviews were typically conducted by phone.

The multiple methodological failures of all of the outcome studies of psychotherapy anticipate a bold conclusion: not one single study survives scrutiny of the contemporary literature of psychotherapy to stand as scientifically credible. Not one study is even a near approximation of convincing research, escaping most of the pitfalls of scientific research in clinical practice. Yet, year in and year out, clinical research protocols are funded by an apparently compliant government in spite of their obvious flaws and, consequently, their obvious inability to resolve their defining problems. It is difficult to avoid the wider conclusion that government's inattention to the methodological pitfalls of psychotherapy's outcome research reflects society's satisfaction with the practice of psychotherapeutics. The following superior examples of contemporary research are organized by the problems they purport to remedy.

The Treatments and Their Outcomes

Depression

Depression and related mood disorders are a major target for psychotherapy; the controlled studies of psychotherapeutic treatments for depression constituted the largest focus of psychotherapeutic outcome research. This is not surprising since the symptoms of mood disorders—unhappiness, despair, feelings of inadequacy, and so forth—are nearly universal and customarily very distressing. Many people seek release from their prolonged depressions; indeed a very large market exists for remedies for unhappiness. In exaggerated, clinical forms, depression and the mood disorders have been implicated in a variety of socially dysfunctional behaviors: withdrawal, torpor, aggression, divorce, child abuse, loss of sleep, unemployment and poor job performance, drug and alcohol dependency, loss of creativity, and so forth.

The field offers the testimony of a series of controlled clinical trials for the efficacy of a variety of treatments for depression: counseling and psychological management; general psychotherapies; short-term and long-term therapies, including cognitive and behavioral treatments, interpersonal psychotherapy, dynamic psychotherapy, and group therapies (TPD 1989, 1728–29). In spite of their different theoretical assumptions about the nature and treatment of depression, many of these psychotherapies seem to be equally effective. This is particularly curious since the combatants in the fierce debate between the two main camps of treatment—the cognitive group and the behavioral group—claim that their underlying assumptions about the causes and treatments for depression are considerably different.

Cognitive therapy, sometimes called cognitive-behavior therapy, is essentially predicated on the assumption that depressed behavior is a result of individuals' distorted views of themselves and their worlds. These negative views of self, interpersonal relations, and the future—Beck's cognitive triad—are activated by "automatic thoughts"; the patient makes "silent assumptions" that the distressing symptoms of depression are the natural and deserved consequences of personal inadequacies. Consequently, cognitive therapy focuses on the factually inaccurate and self-defeating logic—the systematic errors—of the relationship between depressed patients' attributes on the one hand and their emotional and social life on the other. Cognitive therapy attempts to correct these errors through a number of interventions: a process by which the patient monitors his thoughts, a mechanism for evaluating the accuracy of those thoughts, and "homework," that is, exercises for the patient to practice between therapy sessions. This therapeutic process relies upon a belief in the ability of people to change their behaviors through self-reflection and a consequent belief that clinically dysfunctional patients can discipline themselves for cure under the tutelage of a therapist who is trained to judiciously apply the interventions of cognitive therapy. Moreover, cognitive therapy has a rational appeal in that it corrects cognitive misperceptions relative to an objective reality (TPD 1989, chap. 169).

The logic of behavioral therapy is quite different. The behavioralist approach to depression devalues the patient's mental states and ability to reflect upon his or her situation and assumes that dysfunctional symptoms are conditioned responses to negative reinforcements. Depression is a learned response that can be corrected through the appropriate application of learning theory:

> The depressogenic process begins with the occurrence of antecedents of "evoking events." Such stressors initiate the path to a depressive episode to the extent that they disrupt substantial, important, and relatively automatic ("scripted") behavior patterns of individuals. The disruption of these scripted patterns, which constitute typical but crucial aspects of a person's interactions with the environment, produces an initial, immediate negative emotional response (e.g., dysphoria). As a result, the balance of the quality of a person's interactions with the environment (reinforcement) is shifted in a negative direction. (TPD 1989, 1848)

A series of behavioral tactics are at the heart of treatment. These tactics are designed to increase a patient's pleasant interactions (positive reinforcements) with his environment and decrease unpleasant ones (negative reinforcements). A variety of treatments have been developed that focus on concrete as opposed to mental tasks: Lewinsohn's "Coping with Depression Course," social interaction therapy, self-control therapy, social skills training, operant reinforcement, and others.

A study by Miller et al. (1989) that attempted to settle the behavioral-cognitive dispute, and The National Institute of Mental Health Treatment of Depression Collaborative Research Program, which is perhaps the largest psychotherapy research project ever undertaken, are among the best and most frequently cited of the recent research. Their failures to adequately test efficacy signal the state of psychotherapy outcome research generally.

Cognitive versus Behavioral Therapy

Miller et al. (1989) tested three treatment approaches to depressed inpatients. The first, standard treatment, consisted of hospital "milieu" therapy, pharmacotherapy, and medication management sessions with a psychiatrist. These twenty-minute medication sessions occurred once per day while patients were in the hospital and six to eight times during the twenty-week outpatient period. The second treatment condition, cognitive therapy, was provided on top of the standard treatment. It began "after the second week of hospitalization and continued on a once-a-day basis while the patient was in the hospital and for 20 weeks after discharge...typically on a weekly basis...all sessions were 50 minutes in length" (29). The third treatment, social skills training, a behavioral approach, was also provided in addition to the standard treatment, but as an alternative to cognitive therapy, lasting the same amount of time and with the same intensity.

Miller et al. (1989) found that each of their "treatment conditions produced significant improvements at discharge from the hospital and the end of treatment 4 months later" (41). However, by the end of treatment the groups receiving cognitive therapy and social skills therapy in addition to the standard treatment contained patients with fewer and less severe psychiatric symptoms and contained higher percentages of patients who made complete recoveries than did groups of subjects who received the standard treatment alone.

Yet, even from the outset the possibility seems remote that social skills training—or short-term skills training of any type for distressed or very deprived patients—could be effective. People who pass through their youths without acquiring rudimentary social skills are probably not easily educable for a variety of persistent reasons. The notion that their learned incapacities, persisting frequently through many decades of life's challenges, can be simply dispelled through a few sessions of psychotherapeutic training seems naive and too hopeful of socially efficient cures. It seems likely that when simple skills training appears effective it may not have been needed in the first place; the subjects of the research may not have been very debilitated to begin with or the research took advantage of natural learning. Yet, studies without placebo controls cannot fairly test this proposition. For this and many other methodological reasons, not only Miller et al. (1989), but the large accumulated literature of skills training has failed to provide a single credible study to dispel an increasingly justified skepticism.

With unusual candor, Miller et al. (1989) identified four methodological problems with their study: small sample sizes (less than twenty and often less than fifteen); pretreatment differences between samples (e.g., the social skills group contained patients with "a greater degree of personality difficulties"); "only one therapist per psychotherapy was used"; and a lack of uniformity in administering medications.

In addition, the authors might have gone on to emphasize that their study suffered a high rate of attrition (30 percent); the raters "were not blind to the treatment condition nor assessment period"; and the measures were subject to patient and researcher biases. A nontherapy control was not employed, which limits the degree to which experimental outcomes, if they existed, could have been attributed to the two therapeutic conditions. Finally, the authors' own stakes, possibly in behavioral therapy and possibly the unintended source of the positive outcomes themselves, were not considered in the research.

Yet, in spite of these large methodological problems, the authors still insisted that "the results of this study suggest that cognitive-behavioral treatments can produce additional benefits 4 months after discharge for depressed patients who required hospitalization (Miller et al. 1989)." Neither the study itself nor the authors' discussion of their findings put to rest the very live possibility that patients did not improve from therapy. Improvements, if they occurred at all and if they were sustained, were perhaps the result of the simple benefits of periodic surveillance or the cessation of abusive conditions attendant on the patients' decisions to seek therapy. A less complimentary conclusion for psychotherapy keeps intruding itself: the key to treating depressed patients may lie in a nonabusive environment, not in the elegant constructs, rare insights, and skills of trained psychotherapists.

The CRP

Imber et al. (1990), Elkin et al. (1989), and Sotsky et al. (1991) reported the findings of a large-scale experiment conducted on behalf of the federal government: the National Institute of Mental Health Treatment of Depression Collaborative Research Program (CRP). "Two hundred thirty-nine outpatients with major depressive disorder according to the Research Diagnostic Criteria entered a 16-week multi-center clinical trial and were randomly assigned to interpersonal psychotherapy, cognitive-behavior therapy, imipramine with clinical management, or [drug] placebo with clinical management." Interpersonal psychotherapy "focuses on the 'here and now' and relates the patient's depressive condition to a number of areas of interpersonal difficulties: unresolved grief, role transitions, role disputes, and interpersonal deficits" (TPD 1989, 1732).

Reporting on the CRP, Imber et al. (1990) concluded that their "predictions about differential treatment effects were not supported in general" (355) by their large-scale comparison of alternative therapies:

> none of the therapies produced clear and consistent effects at the termination of acute treatment on measures related to its theoretical origins.... [Nevertheless] most patients seen in this program had a successful course of treatment, regardless of modality.... Perhaps the most parsimonious interpretation of our findings is that there are core processes that operate across treatments, overriding differences among techniques, that is, the common factors noted earlier. (356–57)

Unfortunately, their measures were largely based upon self-report; attrition of their samples averaged about 38 percent; inter-rater reliabilities were variable; and success in treatment was not consistent across many measures. Most notably, no true nontreatment control existed for psychotherapy, and only a drug placebo for imipramine. Moreover there was a "general lack of significant differences between the psychotherapies" and the drug placebo group (Elkin et al. 1989).

The study began with 250 patients. Eleven dropped out before treatment. Of the remaining 239 patients, only 155 completed treatment and had complete records. Completion of treatment was defined as attending 75 percent of the sixteen sessions. Moreover, the researchers failed to consider other "core processes" that could have produced their findings, namely, the expectancies of the therapists and researchers, that is, the delicate manner in which their positive hopes for treatment success may have encouraged patients to report nonexistent improvements. It is particularly relevant that those patients who received simply "supportive clinical management," supposedly the least intense of the treatments, fared *better* than the other groups along a variety of scores, most noteworthy, the combined "endogenous" score that measures personal changes, as well as sleep disturbances, appetite changes, psychomotor changes, and so forth. At the end of therapy, 71 percent of the supportive clinical management group did better than the median as compared with only 49 percent of the next most successful group.

If anything, the CRP study suggests that a range of superficial interventions are incapable of producing powerful effects in severely debilitated patients. This would be the common understanding: sixteen weeks of intermittent discussions, even supplemented by drugs that impact directly on mood, are inadequate to sustain improvements in depressed patients. But the authors did not say this, choosing instead to reaffirm the creed of therapy in spite of their own data and porous research methods.

The CRP also reported that "the results of this collaborative clinical treatment trial comparing the efficacy of two specific forms of psychotherapy with active and placebo pharmacotherapy demonstrate the relevance of patient characteristics for the prediction of outcome from an episode of major depressive disorder" (Sotsky et al. 1991). However, the design problems of the study, especially attrition, will not sustain this conclusion. The huge amount of attrition raises the likelihood that subjects self-screened themselves for the therapy most consistent with their own styles. Rather than predicting cure, patient characteristics may simply have predicted the most favored type of ceremony for their own natural remission.

An occasional note of skepticism crept into at least the Elkin et al. (1989) report:

> Further work will be directed toward understanding the therapeutic properties of the PLA-CM condition in the study. The present findings do raise the possibility that some type of minimal supportive therapy in the hands of an experienced practitioner may be sufficient to bring about a significant reduction of depressive symptoms (at least in the short run) for the less severely depressed patients. The findings, if replicated, also raise questions regarding the need of antidepressant medication or for highly specified forms of psychotherapy for the resolution of the depressive episode in these patients.

Perhaps too, all the conditions of treatment and their "core processes," superficial as they were, simply constituted placebo care. Instead of pursuing the obvious inability of short-term therapy to provide gains over a nontreatment control, Elkin et al. (1989) pressed to reinterpret the nontreatment control as true treatment in an attempt to present the findings as universally effective. It is also noteworthy that McLean and Taylor (1992) pointedly failed to corroborate the Elkin et al. (1989) reanalysis.

In spite of a few tortured acknowledgments to skepticism, the CRP reports adopted a pervasive tone of buoyant optimism while their analyses and reanalyses strained to provide evidence of effectiveness. However, their hopeful science was not simply a private venture. It was funded and apparently sanctioned by NIMH, expressing not merely a sectarian bias for positive findings but a deeper social demand, delivered through the federal government, for socially efficient myths, in this case that relatively inexpensive care provides substantial gains against serious depression. The demand for results and reports that support prevailing professional stakes and the expectations of government for politically viable findings are transmitted through funding decisions. Even the peer review process, whether blind or conscious of authorship, that determines which research proposals are funded is open to a variety of institutional, methodological, and reputational biases. It is difficult to avoid the conclusion that this large experiment in treating severe depression became a project in producing compatible findings but not one that provided scientific scrutiny of psychotherapy's clinical effectiveness.

The remainder of the best of the current literature that tested the effects of psychotherapy on depression made similar errors and fell into similar pitfalls of research. Yet, their reported results were consistently positive, testifying to the effectiveness of a variety of treatments in curing depression and related mood disorders. In spite of the fact that the length of therapy seems of have declined over the past few decades—with short-term intervention becoming the treatment of choice and the preference of managed care—outcomes are as rosy now as they were before Smith, Glass, and Miller (1980). Nevertheless, the short-term interventions appear to be so superficial and their controls so inadequate that natural remission—depression being resolved naturally over time—seems as likely a cure as Thompson et al.'s (1987) twenty sessions of bibliotherapy, Nezu and Perri's (1990) ten sessions of problem-solving therapy, McClean and Hakstian's (1990) ten-week courses of nondirective psychotherapy and relaxation therapy, and Lewinsohn et al.'s (1990) fourteen-session "Coping with Depression Course."[3]

Contrary to the optimism of the TPD authors (TPD 1989, 1732–34, 1816–22), the clinical trials of psychotherapy for depression and associated mood disorders have not provided credible proof that any psychotherapeutic treatment is effective. To the contrary, the literature seems content to avoid rigorous tests of outcomes while dressing up the biases of the researchers in the lab coats of science. Neither alternative theories nor alternative treatments have been evaluated. Indeed, the apparently self-serving weaknesses of the tests themselves suggest that even the reported positive outcomes may have been manufactured by the researchers' obvious stakes in their own treatments. It seems equally obvious that society is content with this state of affairs, at least to the extent to which the large subsidies provided by the federal government to this research (usually through NIMH) may reflect a cultural consensus. The curiosity of supposedly different theories that predict similar results exists throughout psychotherapy in tribute to the therapeutic aphorism by Luborsky, Singer, and Luborsky (1975) that everyone is a winner. However, the true conflicts over the different therapeutic approaches may be less over real alternatives and more over prestige and rival commercial interests: Beck, the principal advocate of cognitive-behavioral therapy, is associated with a treatment organization, The Center for Cognitive Therapy, while one of his principal competitors, Lewinsohn, is in the business of marketing his behavioral cure, "The Coping with Depression Course."

Nevertheless, cognitive and behavioral treatment approaches may not be alternatives at all except that each may label its product differently. Lacking a true theoretical distinction or a concrete ability to specify their conditions of therapy, they can be defined and justified in each others' terms. Cognitive states could themselves be conditioned by environment factors and could be the mechanisms for translating social experience into psychological experience. In contrast, the reinforcements of behavioral therapy need to have a cognitive substrate, that is, reinforcements may be internal as well as external. Beck's cognitive treatment processes could be redefined as providing a series of reinforcements, while behavioral contracting is obviously predicated upon assumptions of self-awareness. While the philosophical underpinnings of each approach may have originally been different, their translation into actual psychotherapies may have conflated their different impulses into similar regimens.

In the end, cognitive and behavioral approaches to depression may be essentially the same, generically providing supportive, uplifting hours of attention to unhappy people. This alternative would seem to suggest that the gross hours of treatment, more than any elegance of care, predicts outcomes. Indeed the "core processes" of treatment may simply be the same as placebo care, that is, time-structured activities that provide surveillance for distressed patients. However, these activities need not be provided by the rarified specialists of psychotherapy; Smith, Glass, and Miller (1980) reported identical levels of success for all types of therapists; the level of training has not seemed to affect outcomes, a finding at the center of Dawes' (1994) critique of the field. Moreover, the possibility that placebo treatments are virtually the same as therapeutic outcomes—and there is considerable evidence that this is in fact the case (Prioleau, Murdock, and Brody 1983; Lambert, Weber, and Sykes 1993)—undercuts the claims of psychotherapists to professional standing.

Nevertheless, the studies were not adequately designed to test the effects of psychotherapy on depression, nor were they able to distinguish the differential treatment effects of the two approaches. To the contrary, their methodological shortcomings, obvious at even the stage of their study protocols, and the frank biases of the researchers begin to suggest that psychotherapeutic treatment for depression may actually be ineffective.

Without credible placebos, the appearance of equivalent effectiveness between the variety of treatments is illusory: they may well be equivalently ineffective. Everyone may be a loser. It is also noteworthy that the psychotherapeutic treatments were not tested against a social control, that is, an intervention that directly changed the patient's environment, and therefore, the general value of a psychological approach to depression has not been established. To the contrary, the many social costs of depression might more profitably be addressed by changing noxious economic, political, and physical environments that produce people who have given up on life. However, these sorts of interventions require far greater expenditures than the relatively modest clinical costs for treating depressed patients.

In this sense, the persistently unsuccessful efforts to either find or to test a clinical cure for depression can be recast as a symbolic effort to avoid greater social investments. Indeed, the immaturity of the scholarship of psychotherapy itself—its inability to even test the outcomes of psychotherapy for depression in a manner that can speak to the issue of a treatment's effectiveness—may serve to perpetuate a convenient social myth even while it appears to retard the scientific progress of psychotherapy itself. Moreover, the scientific immaturity of the field also impedes the ability of the society to address its social problems. If psychotherapeutic interventions necessarily fail and if the consequences of depression constitute a serious social problem, then other strategies, far more expensive and socially disruptive, should become live considerations for social policy. Yet, alternative considerations are hindered by misleading research that props up the culture's persistent belief in the efficacy of psychotherapy. The failures of the psychotherapeutic community either to adequately test its treatments for depression or to acknowledge its deficiencies are repeated throughout the literature of psychotherapy.

Agoraphobia, Anxiety, and Panic

Agoraphobia (fear of open places), anxiety, and panic are all related disorders. The TPD insists that in the treatment of these disorders, "clinical experience and experimental research have shown that the most effective procedures are those that rely on systematic [i.e., graded or graduated] in vivo exposure to the feared situations" (TPD 1989, 2029). Graduated *in vivo* exposure "is conducted on a graduated or hierarchical basis so as to confront the patient with his or her feared situations but without evoking" the intense anxiety produced by the intense exposure of "flooding therapy" (TPD 1989, 2029). In summarizing the overall effectiveness of graduated exposure and after acknowledging some of the limitations of the research, the TPD still concludes that treatment routinely confers many benefits: reduction of phobic anxiety, avoidance, and panic; decreases in depression; and improved marital satisfaction (TPD 1989, 2031). At the same time, the TPD also acknowledges the utility of a variety of other treatments: cognitive techniques, psychodynamic therapies, interpersonal therapies, and others. The following three studies represent the best of the research that supports these general conclusions.

Marchione et al. (1987) compared the relative benefits of three different treatments for agoraphobia: cognitive therapy plus graduated exposure, progressive deep muscle relaxation therapy plus graduated exposure (both are behavioral approaches), and graduated exposure alone.

> Treatment consisted of 16 (group) sessions conducted by experienced protocol therapists. All subjects also received cognitive therapy, 90 minutes of graduated in vivo exposure each session and an extensive rationale, emphasizing self-directed exposure and programmed practice in addition to their primary treatment. Subjects also received cognitive therapy, relaxation training or programmed practice. (319)

Marchione et al. (1987) believed that their study

> represents a unique comparative outcome pilot study of combined cognitive-behavioral and physiological-behavioral interventions versus a unitary behavioral treatment for agoraphobia. Overall, the tripartite assessments revealed statistically significant and clinically meaningful repeated measures and outcome effects across behavioral, psychophysiological, cognitive, and self-report response systems. While there were powerful therapeutic effects observed across all conditions, the combined treatments evinced the most potent, rapid and stable patterns and tridimensional improvements, as compared to graduated exposure alone. (326)

Yet these extraordinary claims, only bounded by the caution that their study was a "pilot," are based upon a seriously flawed methodology. All groups contained fewer than *seven* subjects. Attrition across the study was 26 percent. Many measures were based upon patient self-reports and evaluations of audiotaped sessions. No follow-up measures were taken. All treatments proved equally effective although the study did not employ a true nontreatment control.

The use of "independent research associates" to collect data at posttest and to evaluate audiotapes does not protect against the possibility that patient reports transmitted the expectancies of their therapists. Research associates as evaluators may display an exquisite sensitivity to those patients' characteristics at outcome that enhance the therapeutic reputation of their institution or project. These evaluators are not really "independent" of the stakes of the research enterprise, but only uninvolved in therapy per se. It would have been more accurate to describe the study as a case analysis that was poorly protected against researcher biases and that did not control for placebo effects. All of its reported positive effects could simply have been attributed to the research situation itself and not to any true therapeutic outcome.

Butler et al. (1991) compared cognitive behavior therapy with behavior therapy in treating anxiety disorder. Treatment involved twelve individual sessions, each lasting one hour. Three booster sessions were provided after treatment at intervals of two, four, and six weeks. A number of elements were common to both therapies: "giving information about anxiety; explaining the maintenance of symptoms in terms of vicious circles; developing self-management skills and self-reliance through regular practice outside the treatment sessions; and setting the goal that anxiolytic medication should be reduced." In addition, behavior therapy incorporated relaxation techniques and a hierarchy of graded, regular, frequent, and prolonged exposures to the anxiety producing stimuli.

> Only behavioral strategies were used to build confidence. These included planning pleasurable or rewarding activities, resuming activities that had been given up because of demoralization or fatigue, discussing behavior methods for dealing with specific problems and using self-reward and graded task assignment. (Butler et al. 1991)

In contrast, cognitive therapy assumed that anxiety could be controlled by learning to recognize anxious thoughts, to choose "more realistic and helpful alternatives, and to take action to test these in practice" (Butler et al. 1991, 168–69).

Butler et al. (1991) found "a consistent pattern of change supporting the superiority of cognitive-behavioral therapy over behavioral therapy for patients suffering from moderately severe generalized anxiety disorder" (173). This was one of the few studies that demonstrated the superiority of one treatment over another, employed a nontreatment control, and took follow-up measures. Nonetheless, sample sizes were small (under twenty) while data for some of the important conclusions are based upon only 60 percent of the sample. Attrition was over 25 percent in the behavioral therapy group. Only two therapists, seemingly the authors, were employed in the study, and they appear to have been committed to cognitive-behavioral therapy. "Both therapists had originally been trained as behavior therapists, had visited the Center for Cognitive Therapy in Philadelphia for training in cognitive-behavioral therapy, and had used the methods for treating both anxiety and depression" (168). Many of the measures were based upon patient self-report, but some were based upon presumably independent "assessor" ratings via tapes.

But in this study as in many others that utilize audio- and videotapes in an attempt to assure unbiased ratings, the procedures are flawed and compromise the impartiality of the ratings. In checking for treatment integrity, the authors submitted tapes of therapy sessions to "two sets of independent raters... [who] identified the treatments correctly in all the tapes submitted to them. The specific content of the sessions was also rated as clearly different between" the two therapies (170). Presumably then, the independent outcome "assessors" would also have clues that would frequently violate the blinding of a patient's treatment status.

Winston et al. (1991) reported that improvements in the target complaints of patients in their two treatment conditions—short-term dynamic psychotherapy and brief adaptational psychotherapy—were 39 percent and 41 percent, respectively, while the wait-list improved by 18 percent without any treatment, producing a net treatment effect of 21 percent and 23 percent, respectively. If the treatment outcomes are also adjusted by the Lambert, Weber, and Sykes (1993) conservative estimate of the average placebo effect of 16 percent improvement and then adjusted again for the pitfalls of their research—expectancy biases, rater biases, and attrition (presumably a measure of treatment failure)—then differences between treated and untreated groups disappear. Indeed, if these adjustments are reasonable, then time itself (the "treatment" for patients on the wait list) may end up actually being *more* beneficial for people with personality disorders than the "focused interpersonal approach" of the "patient-therapist relationship."[4]

Posttraumatic Stress Disorders

Brom, Kleber, and Defares (1989) compared three different therapies—trauma desensitization, hypnotherapy, and psychodynamic therapy—with a wait-list control in treating "serious disorders resulting from traumatic events (bereavement, acts of violence, and traffic accidents)" (607). The mean number of sessions for hypnotherapy was 14.4; trauma desensitization, 15.0; psychodynamic therapy, 18.8.

The Brom, Kleber, and Defares (1989) study is unusually open and unprotective of the value of its findings. In a manner similar to most of the other outcome studies of psychotherapy, Brom, Kleber, and Defares (1989) could have made the same exaggerated claims for all of their treatment conditions. Because the means of their treated groups showed improvements while those of the wait-list control did not, they concluded that "for psychotherapeutic treatments specifically aimed at posttraumatic stress disorders, this study confirms that which had already been found in general evaluative studies of psychotherapy." However, they pointed out that

> the treatments do benefit some in comparison with a control group and using stringent methodological techniques, but they do not benefit everyone, the effects are not always substantial, and the differences between the therapies are small. Actually,

> clinically significant improvements could be observed in about 60 percent of the treated patients and in 26 percent of the untreated group. The similarity of the results in the three treatment conditions may be due to similarities in the behavior of the therapists, which we did not measure directly; if so, this behavior certainly is based on quite diverging theoretical considerations. (Brom, Kleber, and Defares 1989)

While their caution was commendable, they did not go far enough in questioning alternative explanations for their largely insubstantial findings. Time is itself the most frequent healer of trauma. The possibility of unaided self-healing is particularly pertinent in this study of customarily functional people, most of whom "were in crisis at the time of their application" (608). With this group, remission would be an expected event. But a wait-list control is inadequate to control for time. The denial of therapy may set in motion a number of confounding events, perhaps anger and frustration at being denied quick access to a cultural symbol of understanding and sympathy (therapy). These feelings may inhibit people on the wait-list from acknowledging remission of their trauma and grief. In this case, a nontreatment or placebo control (time-structured activities, perhaps an arts and crafts class, or a discussion with a sports enthusiast) would provide a valuable contrast to formal therapy. Moreover, follow-up measures were not taken with wait-list patients, who were in treatment by that time.

Furthermore, the study does not lay to rest the very plausible idea that its positive findings might well have been due to a temporary adaptation to the treatment situation itself, a response to the tacit demands of therapists for positive (but inaccurate) feedback concerning their care, and the short-lived effect of confrontational techniques. The researchers noted increased patient self-esteem in treated groups. But this might well have resulted from the therapeutic environment that reinforced the implicit expectations of their therapists, perhaps even verbalized as demands, that patients should think better of themselves. This gain is probably transitory even though patients at follow-up may have continued to report what they thought their therapists wanted to hear. Moreover, since the therapies apparently employed unpleasant confrontational techniques, patients may have been reluctant to face more confrontation by reporting their continuing symptoms.

Brom, Kleber, and Defares (1989) note a number of anomalies in their findings, for example, "our conjecture was that short-term psychotherapy would not lead to personality changes. *Some changes in the examined personality characteristics, however, did seem to take place"* (emphasis added). Unfortunately, the paradoxical findings do not lead them into a deeper scrutiny of the research situation (measures, biases, samples, etc.), but into attempts to reconcile their data with psychotherapeutic theory.

Yet they were sufficiently troubled by their findings to acknowledge, although indirectly, the failure of their study to account for its outcomes: "[Our] conclusions make it clear that the process of psychotherapy must be taken into consideration if we want to establish a more explicit link among theory, therapy, research methods, and disorders." In other words, they were not sure that the process of psychotherapy was responsible for their outcomes. Indeed, those outcomes may not have existed; they may have been artifacts of the research situation; they may have reflected only the reports of positive changes; they may have been short lived; and they may have been the result of wait-list frustration that retarded the report of the natural remission of trauma and bereavement in the control group.[5]

Psychotherapy with Children

Psychotherapy has been applied to a variety of psychological problems in children, frequently the antisocial behaviors that underpin the society's concern with juvenile delinquency. Kazdin et al. (1989) randomly assigned antisocial children to one of five therapists and to one of three treatments: "problem-solving skills training, problem-solving skills training with in vivo practice, which included therapeutically planned activities to extend training to settings outside of treatment, or client-centered relationship therapy" (523). All three treatments were provided in twenty-five sessions, each lasting fifty minutes, and administered individually to each child as outpatients and inpatients.

> The bulk of [problem-solving skills training] was devoted to enacting interpersonal situations through role play, where the child applied [steps that had been taught. In vivo practice consisted of] therapeutically planned activities outside of the sessions.... The focus of the [relationship therapy] was on developing a close relationship with the child and providing empathy, unconditional positive regard, and warmth...helping the child to express feelings. (527–8)

The Kazdin et al. (1989) study is theoretically important, speaking generally to the broader problem of juvenile delinquency. They report that their

> results are consistent with other studies on the effectiveness of problem-solving skills in altering behavior in aggressive, antisocial, and impulsive children. The literature is relatively sparse in demonstrations of the effects of cognitive-behavioral treatment with children clinically referred for antisocial behavior. Studies showing effects with clinic samples have reported limitations in the extent to which effects generalize to nontreatment settings, are sustained over time, and place individuals within the normative levels of functions.... In the present study, changes in behavior at home and at school were evident, and the effects were sustained through a 1-year follow-up assessment. However, after treatment, the majority of children remained outside the normative range of functioning on measures of deviance at home and at school. [The skills training treatments] tended to place a greater proportion of children within normative levels than relationship training.... Yet, with one exception, the differences among the three treatment conditions were not significant. (533)

However, the study did not utilize a nontreatment control and cannot account for the amount of remission that might naturally be due to the seasonality of antisocial behaviors or to the aging process itself. The measures, all self-reports of parents, teachers, and children, were potentially reactive to the experimental conditions and the therapists' expectancies. The study, replicating many of the unfortunate characteristics of the second phase of the California Youth Authority experiments of the 1960s and 1970s, curiously fell into many of the same methodological pitfalls that invalidated those experiments (Palmer 1974; Lerman 1975).

The minimal interventions of this study were again insufficient to change antisocial behavior. During the study, that is, while the antisocial children were being supervised to some degree, there was a statistically significant but minor change in their behavior. But when the minimal surveillance provided by the study's therapies—its power as a surrogate for more customary social institutions such as the family and the community—was withdrawn, the children largely reverted to their prestudy patterns of antisocial behavior. Problem-solving skills training, even with *in vivo* experience and relationship training, and especially in the short-term mode of the experiment, are unpromising avenues for treating antisocial behaviors, presumably the precursors if not actually the substance of juvenile delinquency. If this social problem is to be handled, normal conditions of childhood probably need to be provided over extended periods of time to all children. The substitution of relatively inexpensive therapies for the provision of these "normative" conditions does not appear to be effective. Renaming the provision of common, nonabusive, family experiences in the terms of specialized psychotherapy simply clouds the issue of care.

The drift of Kazdin et al.'s (1989) discussion is that more *psychotherapy,* perhaps involving multiple influences, is needed.[6] But the force of the accumulated research in psychotherapy, especially when sifted through a critical analysis, is that other approaches—especially social approaches that seek to replicate customary conditions of participation in important cultural institutions, particularly school and the family—need to be embraced. The occasional discussion is not much of a substitute for the substance of care and the institutional conditions of psychotherapy seem quite inadequate to handle the social nature of personal problems. Psychotherapists are poor social advocates; their professional interests lie elsewhere.

Psychotherapy for Substance Abuse

Few personal problems are as directly related to social damage as substance abuse, particularly alcohol and drug addiction. Any ability to cure or to prevent substance abuse would confer immediate fame on the psychotherapist. However, the long history of attempts to prevent and cure substance abuse have not provided any record of consistent effectiveness. Awareness of the failure of these kinds of programs has rarely been the product of outcome studies. More frequently, the inability to remedy addictive behaviors has simply accumulated in the public's consciousness as the number of current addicts who have been through treatment increases.

Psychotherapeutic interventions—covering the range of individual, group, and family interventions, long- and short-term treatment, inpatient and outpatient, and any number of specific tactical approaches—have consistently failed to cure or prevent substance abuse even while the outcome literature typically exaggerates their effectiveness. Addictive behaviors constitute the paradigmatic case of the resistance of human behavior to planned change strategies. It is also an area in which the accumulated psychotherapy literature expresses the paradigmatic resistance of professional ambitions to acknowledge professional limitations. The outcome studies of psychotherapy have minimized the incorrigibility of addictive behaviors, exaggerating the effectiveness of treatment through a variety of design subterfuges: convenient criteria of cure, convenient samples, imperfect monitoring of continuing drug abuse, imperfect controls, short follow-up, and so forth.

Even the rates of reported cure in the literature, low as they may seem, need to be adjusted by the observation that deviancy in general seems to reduce over time, probably as a simple result of maturation. Outcome tests must control for these effects. Poorly controlled experiments and those that select an older population for treatment will naturally demonstrate greater success than if they had focused on teenagers.

Three prominently published and widely cited studies of treatment success are among the best studies in the field. It is noteworthy that each one provides a relatively inexpensive intervention; each one claims success; and each one seems to cross the border between allowable inferences from their data into willfully misleading research. All of the design problems of these studies should have either been anticipated and corrected or clearly acknowledged in the write-up of findings.

Miller (1980) randomized problem drinkers, 88 percent of them self-referred, to a bibliotherapy control and three treatment conditions: self-control training involving six weekly sessions; self-control training "plus 12 sessions of relaxation, communication, and assertion training; or, self-control plus 12 weeks of individually tailored broad spectrum" behavior therapy (590).

The Miller (1980) findings are particularly suggestive:

> The present findings replicate results of previous research indicating no significant differences in effectiveness between minimal [self-control training] and more extensive interventions for problem drinkers.... Bibliotherapy clients showed less improvement on one sensitive change measure, the number of hours per week intoxicated.... The fact that [these clients] were starting from a significantly higher level of self-reported alcohol consumption at in-take must be considered in interpreting this difference. On other measures of alcohol consumption and of functioning on non-drinking dimensions, no differences among groups were found. *The total improvement rate of 60 percent [for the bibliotherapy control group] compares favorably with comparable rates from the other groups. Thus bibliotherapy, although not excelling in absolute effectiveness, appears to be a relatively cost-effective procedure.* (599, emphasis added)

The particular methodological problems of this study—small samples (approximately twelve), high attrition (27 percent), failure to adjust for seasonality, and self-reported outcome measures—epitomize the failures of psychotherapeutic outcome research to accurately reflect the true experience of therapy.

Miller (1980) presents the communal problem of research in the social services in a nutshell: the researchers fail to discover differences between their two interventive conditions while insisting that the older intervention (in this case, bibliotherapy) is a standard treatment control, and not a nontreatment control or a placebo control. Thus, their findings of equivalence instead of representing negative results are converted by convenient redefinition into a positive finding of cost effectiveness. If bibliotherapy is a treatment control, then both conditions are effective; if a nontreatment control or a placebo, then both are ineffective.

The problems of self-report are debilitating for the research. Addicts are notoriously unreliable and without physical evidence of abstinence, their responses *must* be viewed skeptically, as gaming behavior. Miller (1980) tried to employ a physical test of abstinence, an *in vivo* breath test, at follow-up, but

> although all clients had consented to the procedure, only 17 (out of 41) granted permission when actually contacted for a test at 10 months following termination. Of the remainder, 14 refused the test, 6 had moved out of the area, and 4 were not located. (599)

This forcefully raises the issue of the accuracy of all self-reported "improvements." The study's finding that bibliotherapy can change the behaviors of problem drinkers is also highly fanciful without a nontreatment comparison that is different from bibliotherapy. It is more reasonable to reinterpret the total improvement rate of 60 percent as a suspect placebo effect for self-selected and presumably motivated problem drinkers. This motivation may even explain the distortion of their self-reports. Indeed, the reported 60 percent improvement rate begins to suggest the size of the biases of researchers, their need for positive results, and the degree to which they are prepared to uncritically accept numbers that support their interests.

Miller (1980) found that self-concept, largely self-reported by patients, improved through treatment but did not predict treatment success, which tended to be measured more objectively. Nevertheless, "self-concept may be a very useful index of treatment success and one that fits into the multiple-criteria model of recovery currently being espoused by most researchers" (Miller 1980, 1092). Yet, most people who are not alcoholism therapists and researchers would probably tend to consider reduced drinking or abstinence—not an improved self-concept—as the overwhelmingly important success criteria for the treatment of alcohol addiction.

Woody, McLellan, and Luborsky (1987) wished to settle

> the long-debated issue of the value of psychotherapy as an addition to paraprofessional counseling services for opiate addicts receiving methadone maintenance.... Subjects were randomly assigned to receive either supportive-expressive psychotherapy plus drug counseling, cognitive-behavioral psychotherapy plus drug counseling, or paraprofessional drug counseling alone. Therapy was offered once a week for 24 weeks.... The subjects were male veterans who were addicted to opiates and who were starting a new period of treatment with methadone maintenance (590–91).

Woody, McLellan, and Luborsky (1987) apparently felt that they settled the issue of the effectiveness of psychotherapy with opiate addicts:

> The results from our analysis of baseline to 12-month follow-up were similar to those previously reported for 7-month analyses. All treatment groups showed improvements. However, the two psychotherapy groups showed more improvements than the drug counseling group over a wider range of outcome measures, with marked changes in the areas of employment, legal status, and psychiatric symptoms and with less use of psychotropic medications.
>
> Although the combined data indicate substantial improvement, they do not indicate that the drug addiction was "cured" by psychological treatments, if the term "cured" is defined as the complete cessation of all drug use. However, it is important to note that improvements in areas such as drug use, employment, legal status, and psychiatric status are meaningful in economic and social terms, not only to the patient but to the patient's family, employer and the community. (595)

Yet, the findings are not credible. Except for psychiatric symptomatology, Woody, McLellan, and Luborsky (1987) relied for all of their information on self-reports. They made no independent assessments of any of the responses, not even in areas in which hard measures were possible (urinalysis for drug use, checks on employment, and so forth). Heroin addicts are decidedly not reliable informants relative to their addiction. Their gaming behavior is very sensitive to their perceptions of their benefits in any situation. The researchers instituted no protections against unreliable reports nor against another powerful threat to the validity of the study: the addicts in therapy may have been more motivated to fulfill the therapists "expectations" of cure through inaccurate verbal reports than the addicts in drug counseling. The samples were small, all under thirty-four. While the follow-up evaluations were "done by trained and experienced research technicians who had no role in the treatment," the addicts were quite conscious of the status of their therapists. The psychotherapists represented greater authority than the paraprofessional drug counselors.

In the end, the reports by the addicts may have reflected their different perceptions of the abilities of their therapists to satisfy their needs. Again, no objective tests (in this case urinanalysis) were made to validate the self-reports of the addicts. The addicts may have fulfilled the expectations of their therapists by giving psychiatrists positive reinforcement on psychological variables and providing drug counselors positive reinforcement on addiction measures. In addition, many of the differences were small while the three treatment groups differed at baseline in important ways. The nonpsychotherapy, drug-counseling group had far better employment characteristics than the other two groups. Moreover, it is startling and largely ignored by the researchers, that the nontherapy, drug-counseling group—presumably the control—was the only group to greatly reduce their drug-taking behavior from twelve days of illicit drug use to three days. One psychotherapy group did not change; the other went from four days to two days.

Furthermore, attrition may have been a problem. While the study started with 120 patients, only ninety-three (attrition of 22.5 percent) were available for twelve-month comparisons, and only eighty-four (attrition of 30 percent) were available for the check point at seventeen months. Especially with addicts, the assumption of random or unbiased attrition is not plausible.

Botvin et al. (1990) conducted a large-scale test of drug abuse prevention. Fifty-six schools, containing 4,466 children, in New York State were randomly assigned to three conditions: a prevention program with formal training and implementation feedback, a prevention program with videotaped training, and a condition of "no feedback," that is, no treatment. The prevention program, the Life Skills Training Program (LST),

> consists of 12 curriculum units designed to be taught in 15 class periods. Each unit consists of a major goal for the unit, measurable student objectives, content and classroom activities. LST is designed to be offered to seventh graders.... The main purpose of the LST program is to facilitate the development of personal and social skills, with particular emphasis on the development of skills for coping with social influences to smoke, drink, or use drugs. The LST program teaches students cognitive-behavioral skills for building self-esteem, resisting advertising pressure, managing anxiety, communicating effectively, developing person relationships, and asserting one's rights. These skills are taught using a combination of teaching techniques including demonstration, behavioral rehearsal, feedback and reinforcement, and behavioral "homework" assignments for out of class practice.
>
> In addition...the LST program teaches problem-specific skills and knowledge related to smoking, drinking, and drug use. (439)

The entire prevention program was delivered in fifteen sessions, at the rate of two per week during 1985, and "boosted" with one session in each of the following two years. This is the epitome of the socially efficient promise—important goals (skills for success and the prevention of drug abuse), realized through specialized professional expertise (demonstration, behavioral rehearsal, etc.), that can be achieved within the existing structure (of curriculum in this case) and with little fuss, bother, or pain—just fifteen sessions. LST is a commercially available prevention program. Botvin et al. (1990) found

> additional support for the effectiveness of a cognitive-behavioral approach to substance abuse prevention among junior high school students. Prevention effects were found for cigarette smoking, immoderate alcohol use, and marijuana use. Because their prevention approach was originally developed to reduce adolescent cigarette smoking, it is not surprising that the strongest effects were for smoking... this study provides the largest and most rigorous test of the LST approach and demonstrates the effectiveness of this prevention strategy when ongoing intervention activities are provided throughout the critical junior high school period... the results of this study indicate that even with a modest level of implementation completeness, this prevention approach is capable of producing an impact on drug use. (444)

Botvin et al.'s (1990) conclusions are based upon two types of results, one relating to the self-reported behavior of substance abuse and the other related to the self-reported attitudes, knowledge, skills, and expectations related to substance abuse. The behaviors are the critical outcomes of prevention; the internal states are presumably mediating mechanisms that can be modified in order to prevent or lessen abuse of targeted substances.

With large samples, such as those in this study, extremely small differences will be statistically significant. Yet Botvin et al. (1990) found no significant differences between the experimental groups and the control group in drinking frequency and amount. Small but statistically significant differences were found relative to smoking; very small but still significant differences were found relative to drunkenness and marijuana use. The largest differences—between the control and experimental groups related to smoking—covered only 1.7 percent of the possible range of scores. On a ten-point scale of cigarette smoking (one=never; ten=more than one pack per day), one experimental group scored 1.46; the other experimental group scored 1.50; and, the control scored 1.63. In other words, all groups scored between one ("never" using cigarettes) and two ("not using cigarettes in the past twelve months"). The highest means (around 3, "a few times in the past twelve months") were reported for alcohol use. As noted, the experiment made no impact at all on alcohol use.

With no practical or important impacts on targeted *behaviors,* the *attitudinal* findings become irrelevant. They are also consistently tiny.

All of the Botvin et al. (1990) measures of outcomes were based upon the self-reports of the students. The study did not verify any of these data against objective tests. Their "bogus pipeline" procedure for collecting breath samples at the pretest "in an effort to enhance the validity of substance use self-reports" was not repeated at the posttest (440).

All of the differences are so small that it seems reasonable, perhaps likely, that they can be accounted for simply by stereotypical "goodness" responses among young adolescents who are prodded by fifteen sessions of pep talks. The differences, small and unimportant as they are, may reflect the inability of the intervention to affect even the verbal reports of behaviors of deep concern.

The study itself offers two cautions in interpreting the results: first, "the population for this study consisted of predominantly white, middle-class, suburban and rural students" and "second, this and other school-based studies have consistently found higher attrition among substance users." The study suffered a 25 percent attrition rate. Against the backdrop of the study's methodological deficiencies, its importance could only be demonstrated by large differences between groups, differences that eclipsed the possibility of stereotypical reporting behavior, attrition, and the nonrepresentativeness of the sample. The real test of the Botvin et al. (1990) intervention—LST—should not take place in the favored suburbs, but in the South Bronx. In the end, Botvin et al. (1990) proved nothing except that LST was fundamentally ineffective, chasing imagined problems with superficial cures.

The study, however, is not simply an instance of Barnumlike exaggeration; it tends to support important social myths, in this case, that drug abuse prevention is cheaply obtained. By inference, this suggests too that the real problems of substance abuse in poorer communities are similarly amenable to inexpensive cures. This devalues the far more reasonable claim that if the children of poverty were to be provided with an environment similar to that of the Botvin et al. (1990) sample, then they would manifest a similarly low pattern of abusing behaviors. But the provision of this kind of environment would vastly exceed the comfortably budgeted costs of fifteen sessions of LST. The Botvin study is experimental theater, not science.[7]

Miscellaneous Problems

Anorexia Nervosa

Hall and Crisp (1987) investigated psychotherapy in the treatment of anorexia nervosa. Their therapy group received twelve one-hour sessions of psychotherapy at one- and two-week intervals.

> In each case attention was focused on the role anorexia nervosa played in the relationship of the subject with her family and others. An attempt was made to change those aspects of relationships which tended to stifle the subject's development and maintain the anorexia, particularly over-protectiveness, conflict, avoidance, enmeshment, and distancing within the family. (186)

Hall and Crisp (1987) found that both psychotherapy and dietary advice provided help for patients with anorexia nervosa. They argued that

> it is simplistic to focus on weight gain and the return of menstruation alone as indicators of improvement in anorexia nervosa, and that intrapsychic and interpersonal conflicts, sexual and social adjustment, and continuing development are at least as important. This study demonstrates that significant improvement in overall functioning, as reflected in the global clinical scores, may have been achieved by two different brief interventions.

Nevertheless, weight loss and the suppression of menstruation are the dominant clinical reasons why anorexia nervosa is a problem. The social aspects of the disease have not been implicated as causal elements. The study did not demonstrate the superiority of psychotherapy in restoring weight that was objectively measured; indeed the dietary advice group gained more weight.

The psychotherapy group did show its superiority on measures of sexual and social adjustment. Notwithstanding the authors' preferences, these findings could be reasonably interpreted as secondary or peripheral relative to anorexia nervosa. Moreover, the sexual and social improvements of subjects were rated on the basis of self-reports at follow-up "by an assessor who was blind to the treatment allocated" (Hall and Crisp 1987, 185). However, true blinding seems unlikely; patients and their families probably cued the *single* assessor by either naming the therapist or by referring to some defining characteristic of their treatment. Again, the expectancies of psychotherapists may have been more effectively transmitted to patients through the personal relationships of psychotherapy, than the expectancies of dietary therapists. Moreover, a number of patients in the psychotherapy group seem to have deteriorated. Each group contained only fifteen patients.

In a later study, Crisp et al. (1991) randomized ninety anorectic subjects to one of four treatment groups: inpatient care, outpatient individual and family psychotherapy with dietary counseling, group psychotherapy with dietary counseling, and no further treatment. The inpatient treatment was intensive, involving a stay of several months; "treatment involved weight restoration...supported by weekly individual therapy, family therapy, group therapy, dietary counselling and occupational therapy," followed by twelve sessions of outpatient care. The outpatient individual/family therapy condition involved twelve sessions, "which always addressed the developmental psychopathology, with the focus on its expression immediately preceding the illness onset." The third treatment condition, outpatient group therapy, covered ten sessions for the anorectic patients and ten separate sessions for their families. Patients who received no further treatment were simply referred back to their family physicians.

Crisp et al. (1991) concluded that all of their three interventions to treat anorexia nervosa—inpatient care and two types of outpatient treatments—"are powerful in their effect at one-year follow-up." However, the samples were small and the findings were modest while the authors concede a number of methodological problems that permit alternative interpretations of the outcomes. "This study has been fraught with difficulties that relate to the well known problem of engaging and maintaining patients with anorexia nervosa in treatment and follow-up." Noncompliance was a considerable problem, especially large with the inpatient group, while the outpatient interventions were very brief. Yet, all the treatment groups made progress. In light of the authors' further acknowledgment that the assessment procedure itself may have contaminated the findings, it is difficult to attribute the outcomes to psychotherapy and not simply to the process of surveillance. The fact of periodic and predictable attention given to the patients through their scheduled assessments may have had more effect on weight gain than any form of therapy. While the outpatient groups did best on average, they also contained the patients with the worst outcomes, one who died, and two who became binge eaters. The binge eaters perversely contributed a disproportionate amount of weight gain to the good outcomes of the group. Treatment integrity itself was a problem with the outpatient groups, implying that outpatient care was very superficial and, therefore, a questionable factor in the groups' improvements; group therapy outpatient subjects only attended an average of five out of their ten scheduled sessions; the other outpatient group missed 25 percent of twelve sessions. Furthermore, the poor record of the nontreated control might be more a tribute to the rebuff of the experiment—neglect—than to any sort of typical baseline behavior. Without a true placebo in which the nontreated group believes it is receiving treatment and that controls for attention itself both in the context of therapy and of assessment, the effects of psychotherapy itself are impossible to gauge.

Bulimia

In a similar study that employed a randomized design, Mitchell et al. (1990) compared intensive group therapy and drug therapy in reducing bulimia. The intensive group therapy, provided over nine weeks, focused on the use of behavioral and cognitive behavioral techniques. In its first phase patients met for two two-hour sessions for two weeks. During the second phase subjects met for five three-hour sessions during the first week and then gradually reduced the number of meetings to two over the next three weeks. The final phase provide 1.5-hour meetings once each week to stabilize behaviors.

Mitchell et al. (1990) report large positive results for their randomized evaluation of treatment for bulimia:

> In our current study, in the two psychotherapy cells, we found a mean percent reduction in binge eating of 89% and 92%.... 51% of the subjects were free of bulimic symptoms for the last 2 weeks of treatment, and an additional 35% averaged one or fewer episodes per week during the same period. This suggests that the group intervention was powerful in suppressing and, in many cases, completely interrupting the bulimic pattern.

The authors are unusually candid in acknowledging the principal impediment to the accuracy of their findings:

> The key variables in this report concern eating behavior, and the eating data rest solely on the subjects' self-reports. This reliance on self-reports remains a major limitation to research in this area. Researchers working with this population know

> that, at times, these subjects are untruthful.... It is possible that those subjects in group therapy may have been more likely than those subjects receiving medication alone to misrepresent the degree of their recovery, given the group pressure to be successful.

Indeed, it seems likely that group treatment subjects relayed the expectancies of their therapists and groups. Moreover, true attrition in their research was almost 50 percent; 218 entered the study; only 171 of these lasted to the randomization stage and only 115 finished treatment. While the clinician evaluators were blind to whether patients received placebo drugs or imipramine, they were aware of the patients who were in group treatment. Thus, the clinician evaluators were placed in the suspect position of evaluating the progress of their own patients and by implication their own professional skill. Once again, there was no nontreatment control for group treatment. Finally, there was no follow-up. These faults in the research do not simply recommend caution; they vitiate the findings.[8]

Sexual Abuse

Alexander et al. (1989) compared two different group treatments—interpersonal transaction and a process group—for women who had been sexually abused as children. Groups met for 1.5 hours each week for ten weeks.

> In the interpersonal transaction group format, the therapists introduced a new dyadic disclosure topic each week. Topics focused on issues common to the experience of incest (such as feelings of being different, positive and negative perceptions of self, feelings of helplessness, issues of trust, family secrets, and ambivalence toward mother and father), with a gradual progression across the course of therapy in the intimacy level of weekly topics. Emphasis was placed on the nonjudgmental, sharing common experiences and feelings relevant to the incest and to the family experience.
>
> [In the process group], members shared their goals and expectations as well as their incest histories. Following the recommendations of Yalom (1975), the groups then moved largely to a focus on each member's actual interaction with the group as a means of developing a new perspective on incest, of understanding the problematic interpersonal behaviors that helped perpetuate the member's general "victimization," and of experimenting with new ways of relating to the group, and by extension, people in general. (481)
>
> ...the first empirical data supporting the efficacy of time-limited group therapies as treatments for adult survivors of childhood incest. Both group formats were effective relative to the wait-list condition in reducing depression and in alleviating distress.... Furthermore these changes were maintained at follow-up 6 months

later. It is important to note, however, that subjects were not precluded from being involved in individual therapy following the posttreatment evaluation. Therefore it is possible that the 6-month follow-up data also reflect the influence of subsequent individual therapy.

However, in this study, as in many others, it is not clear what is being treated. The selection criteria for the group was reported sexual abuse. Many of the subjects also suffered a variety of symptoms. But neither the literature nor the researchers have established a causal relationship between sexual abuse and those specific clinical symptoms, nor did the researchers establish the accuracy of sexual abuse claims. It is certainly plausible that the large amount of public media attention paid to incest and other forms of sexual abuse within the family may have encouraged disturbed people and those who pursue therapy recreationally to have imagined or fantasized sexual abuse in order to qualify as subjects in the research. The large number of subjects who went on to individual therapy is also suggestive.

In any event, the findings were not uniformly positive. The greatest gains were made against depression. Treatment groups were small (sixteen and twenty). Moreover, the data, as is common, were based upon patient self-reports to the Beck Depression Inventory.

Nonchronic Schizophrenia

Frank and Gunderson (1990) reanalyzed data from a previous study (Stanton et al. 1984) that assessed the relative value of exploratory-insight-oriented psychotherapy and reality-adaptive-supportive psychotherapy in the treatment of nonchronic schizophrenia. Stanton et al. (1984) had suffered debilitating attrition rates (33 percent from treatment and 50 percent by follow-up) and in the end produced equivocal findings that did not seem to argue for the value of individual psychotherapy in the treatment of their schizophrenic patients. Frank and Gunderson (1990) attempted to evaluate whether the relationship between the therapist and patient, and not the therapy itself, would predict patient success.

Frank and Gunderson (1990) found that "as predicted, patients who formed stronger alliances in the first 6 months of treatment made more gains in more areas during the 2-year study period than patients who did not." Once again, although the findings were statistically significant they were small. However, the study design was inadequate to support its conclusions. Patients who improved during therapy may have been more capable of establishing appropriate relations with their therapists than patients who did not improve. The alliance may not have been the reason for cure but the reverse, that is, the result of improvement, part of the ceremony of cure. Reports of patient improvement from the therapist may have been associated with reports of the patient's increased ability to relate normally. The patients were taking antipsychotic medication along with their psychotherapy and the possibility remains strong that the small amount of improvement was simply associated with medication or time. As the authors report, "consistent with what had been hypothesized, the development of a good alliance was associated with greater acceptance of pharmacotherapy as well as psychotherapy." The confusion of cause and effect in correlational analyses is a fundamental flaw of interpretation.

As is common in large social experiments, the data are reanalyzed to explore alternative hypotheses. However, these reanalyses, especially when they defy the experimental logic of randomization by conflating patients into a single group, do not retain the methodological power of the original design. While reanalyses can be valuable in pointing to new possibilities for treatment, those possibilities need to be retested in experiments that are specifically controlled for the new hypotheses. The Frank and Gunderson (1990) reanalysis did not do this even while it retained all of the design imperfections of the original Stanton et al. (1984) experiment.

Pilkonis et al. (1984) compared three different treatment approaches—individual, conjoint, and group psychotherapy—for outpatients suffering from

> an affective, anxiety, adjustment, or personality disorder; and be living with another adult who would be willing to act as an informant, and, if necessary, to agree to participate in conjoint therapy.... Treatment was provided by experienced private clinicians who valued highly the specific form of therapy they provided. (432)

The mean number of sessions was 26.8, normally scheduled for weekly psychiatric hours, with no significant differences among the three approaches. Pilkonis et al. (1984) reported that

> although our purpose was to compare the relative effectiveness of individual, group, and conjoint therapy, the most notable finding was the clinically significant improvement of the sample as a whole. Even more impressive than the generally

> positive outcomes at termination was the maintenance of these gains at the follow-up evaluation, after a posttreatment period that averaged 31 weeks. The consistent and stable improvement among our patients was probably due, in part, to the quality and experience of the therapists, whose mean age was 45 years and who had an average of 11 years of experience.

The alternative explanation is less flattering to the skill of the therapists. The skill of clinicians may well lie largely in their ability to establish enduring, pleasant relationships with clients and not in any therapeutic capacity. No independent or objective measures were taken; patients, their significant others, and the therapists themselves, selected because of their commitment to particular modes of therapy, rated patient outcomes in the treatments that they provided. Samples were small (twenty-one and twenty-two). Randomization was consciously breached by the experimenters in one third of the cases because of the slow initial recruitment of patients.

Attrition was an enormous problem, producing a test sample that cannot be generalized to any population. Of the initial group of ninety-two study patients, seven dropped out of the study before their first interview (8 percent attrition), and sixteen dropped out before completing 6 sessions of therapy (25 percent attrition). Five additional patients refused to provide any information for evaluations (30 percent total attrition for posttest evaluation), and eight more were lost between the end of therapy and the follow-up (40 percent total patient attrition). Attrition of significant others was even higher (46 percent total attrition). The attrition rates are yet higher if the study base is considered to be the eighty-five who started therapy instead of the ninety-two who were initially recruited.

There is a curious lack of data provided by the study about specific group outcomes and interrater reliabilities, especially since the authors note that interrater "correlations within informants tended to be stronger than correlations across informants (even though the same instruments were sometimes rated)" (Pilkonis et al. 1984, 433).

The study did not employ a nontreatment control, which prevents attributing outcomes to the therapies themselves. In this regard, they reported a number of background factors (e.g., social class) that are unrelated to therapy per se, but that predict success in therapy. Instead of assuming that these factors are associated with therapeutic receptivity, it might be equally reasonable to assume that they provide the inherent ability for self-cure.

Headache and Hypertension

Holroyd and Andrasik (1982) report statistically significant differences between cognitive therapy and biofeedback in the treatment of headache two years after treatment. "Wolcoxon matched-pairs and signed-ranks test revealed that headache sufferers who received stress-coping training recorded fewer headaches, fewer hours of headache, and less overall headache activity...at the two year follow-up (p less than .005)" (330). But the critical comparison—underlying the point of the study that stress coping is superior to biofeedback—lies in the sustained overall group differences between stress coping and biofeedback. These differences were not computed by the researchers, perhaps because the sustained improvement of those who received biofeedback (four of eight) and those who received stress coping (nine of eleven) is not statistically significant (Fisher exact test, p=.175). Without a discussion of this outcome the study itself is very misleading. It prevents the authors from reaching their extended conclusion that stress-coping training

> may prove of value in the management of disorders other than headache. The theoretical rationale for this approach to the treatment of stress related illness has been outlined by Holroyd (1979). (Holroyd and Andrasik 1982)

Biofeedback may actually be a good nontreatment control, a true placebo, and not an alternative treatment.

In addition, the pretreatment differences between their very small samples (eight and eleven) are large, although not statistically significant, on measures of headache severity (e.g., 5.4 headaches per week in the cognitive group versus 7.0 in the biofeedback group). These differences challenge the value of the outcomes. Once again, the researchers' discussion should have included an analysis of the degree to which the pretreatment differences, instead of stress-coping training, may have accounted for the sustained outcomes of the research.

Hypertension

Tosi et al. (1992) randomly assigned subjects to three different treatment regimens for reducing mild-to-moderate hypertension and to an attention placebo. All subjects went through seventy-five-minute sessions once a week for eight weeks. Those assigned to cognitive restructuring and hypnosis were exposed to a variety to audiotapes, readings, and cognitive restructuring exercises (e.g., the Harvard Group Hypnotic Susceptibility tape, two "30-minute tapes that incorporated hypnosis and cognitive restructuring, a tape recording of Albert Ellis's Rational Emotive Therapy"). In this experiment cognitive restructuring emphasized "the restructuring of irrational ideas, attitudes, and beliefs theoretically and empirically associated with hypertension." Patients in the hypnosis group were only exposed to the hypnosis tapes. Patients in the cognitive restructuring group only received the cognitive restructuring material. Placebo subjects "participated in weekly discussions with the facilitator and addressed issues pertaining to medication, career pressure, roles, and life plans." All sessions were lead by one "advanced Ph.D. counseling student who was trained in hypnosis and cognitive restructuring" (Tosi et al. 1992).

Tosi et al. (1992) pick through their very equivocal outcome data to produce an optimistic series of findings. "[T]he overall multivariate model consisting of all experimental conditions over time yielded a significant effect with respect to nine psychobiological outcome measures." Moreover, they report that the group that received both cognitive restructuring and hypnosis did best. However, the principal outcome criteria, blood pressure, dropped only slightly while the placebo group also demonstrated gains. The study's credibility is further harmed by its very small samples, ranging from seven to eleven subjects, and the fact that all treatment groups were lead by a single "facilitator." Some of the outcome measures were objective (e.g. systolic blood pressure). However, many of the outcomes were reported through patient questionnaires that asked about anxiety, aggression, and anger and were obviously susceptible to the lone facilitator's expectancy biases. Tosi et al. (1992) make much of isolated outcome occurrences, ignoring the great variability of their data. In spite of their claims, there is little to recommend any of their treatments.

Culturally Sensitive Therapy

Malgady, Rogler, and Costantino (1990) reported on two experiments in providing culturally sensitive therapy to prevent mental disorder among Puerto Rican children. In the first experiment, 210 Puerto Rican children, who were rated as behavioral problems by their parents and teachers and, therefore, "classified in the secondary prevention stage for risk of mental disorder," were randomly assigned to two treatment conditions ("cultural intervention sessions") and two controls. For the first treatment condition,

> a panel of Puerto Rican psychologists and parents selected 40 cuentos [fables] with child protagonists from Puerto Rican folklore on the basis of thematic content embodying cultural values. [The second treatment condition], consistent with the bicultural approach, was developed by adapting these cuentos to bridge Puerto Rican and American cultures and to convey more therapeutically the moral of each story. The ethnic identity of the main character remained Puerto Rican in the adapted stories, but other characters were presented as multiethnic (Hispanic, Black, and White) to more naturally reflect inner-city social interactions.

The first of the treatment controls was an art/play therapy group that employed "recreational tasks and games in which mother-child dyads interacted under the supervision of a therapist." A second control received no therapy at all and simply participated in discussion sessions lead by a therapist and a school teacher. All of the conditions were provided in twenty weekly, ninety-minute sessions.

The second experiment employed group sessions with ninety Puerto Rican eighth and ninth graders who were also judged to be at risk of mental disorder. This time the stories presented "heroic" role models drawn out of Puerto Rican history. The adolescents were randomly assigned to the hero/heroine therapy group that went through eighteen weekly, ninety-minute sessions or to an attention control group that participated in eight monthly discussion sessions.

Malgady, Rogler, and Costantino (1990) reported mixed results in their two experiments to prevent mental disorder among Puerto Rican children through culturally sensitive therapy. In the first experiment, "treatment effects were significant in the analyses of anxiety symptoms, social judgment, and aggression observation ratings; however, differential treatment outcomes were not evident in disruptive behavior, delay of gratification, or self-concept." In the second experiment utilizing hero/heroine therapy with Puerto Rican adolescents, only one of the results, and this relatively unimportant, was significant. However, the authors conclude that "the findings of the cuento and hero/heroine research show that cultural interventions produced generally more favorable outcomes than did no-treatment intervention, lending support to the conclusion that cultural match or mismatch is indeed consequential."

Yet, the few statistically significant findings, largely in the first experiment, were very small, a result of the large samples, and arguably of little practical or theoretical importance. Moreover, the small gains are themselves suspect since it seems unlikely that the interviewers were consistently blind to the group status of the subjects, especially those who were enrolled in the nontreatment control. However, the authors completely ignored the social conditions that may have provoked their subjects' antisocial behavior, preferring instead to dwell on a psychotherapeutic strategy for achieving cultural adaptation.

A more accurate summary of their very minimal psychological approach to the behavioral problems of poor children would have interpreted the experiments as failures. With greater cultural sensitivity for the futures of those children, the authors might have pointed to their needs for family supports including jobs and income for their parents, better schools, and more hospitable communities. However, this latter would cost far more than a few story-telling sessions for school children. Without a sense of the deprivation of poor Puerto Rican children in New York City, their belletristic interventions were doomed from the start. It seems a mockery of cultural sensitivity for psychotherapy research to so completely ignore the true social and economic deficits of children in self-absorption with its narrow professional concern: "what type of psychotherapy administered by whom is most effective for which type of client with what type of problem under which set of circumstances?" (Malgady, Rogler, and Costantino 1990, quoting Paul).[9]

Conclusion: The State of Psychotherapy Knowledge

The psychotherapy outcome literature prior to 1980 could not sustain the happy conclusion that the field was capable of treating any psychological problem. Aside from its numerous methodological deficiencies, the Smith, Glass, and Miller (1980) review failed to rigorously evaluate the quality of the many studies that constituted their base of evidence; they relied upon research that was biased, inappropriately controlled and uncontrolled, poorly analyzed, theoretically trivial, unreliable, and deficient in other regards. Subsequent to 1980, the outcome evidence for the effectiveness of individual and group psychotherapy will still not sustain any conclusion of effectiveness and for the same reasons. In spite of a greater number of randomized studies, the base of research is still deficient and in largely the same ways: small samples, biased measures and unreliable measurement, self-serving and inappropriate analyses, and so forth. At best the effectiveness of psychotherapy remains indeterminate. Indeed, the poor quality of the primary clinical tests of effectiveness, uncorrected and still immature after many decades of effort, is more suggestive of a pseudoscientific endeavor than a true scientific enterprise. Most of the recent summaries of the field have repeated Smith, Glass, and Miller's (1980) mistakes, accepting largely at face value the convergence of bulk-cargo studies and failing to ground their observations in the quality of the research that produced the data. As a result, reported findings and conclusions are customarily positive. They constitute the wisdom of psychotherapy, enacted in the mantra of textbooks, summary works, collections, reviews, and treatment manuals.

With almost no chance of producing credible findings, an ethical issue is raised about flawed studies: Why were subjects pestered and resources expended on hopelessly flawed exercises? The answer may lie in the mythic value of their testimony to the ability of relatively inexpensive interventions to bring about greater happiness and social adjustment among American citizens and largely through their own initiative in solving their own personal problems. These sorts of studies are acts in the drama of the helping hand, but they are not credible clinical science.

The field's roseate affection for its mission has blunted the development of a truly rigorous research community. Even the field's few critics frequently sidestep the lack of empirical validation to press alternative but still untested theories of treatment. Among the few dissenters, most have been loyal critics seemingly satisfied to perennially identify the correctable deficiencies of the field's scholarship while implicitly assuming that the weight of common clinical experience will eventually sustain the effectiveness of treatment without the necessity for sophisticated scientific scrutiny of outcomes. Few have been willing to consider that psychotherapy is a pseudoscience in pursuit of a pseudocure.

The quality of research in family therapy gives even greater weight to the evaluation of psychotherapy as pseudoscience. The deficiencies of individual and group psychotherapy are even more evident in the emergent psychotherapeutic specialty of family treatment. Just like its parent field, family therapy fails to offer any credible proof of its effectiveness.

Notes

1. The following randomized studies were omitted from the analysis simply because their invalidating inadequacies were redundant with the studies that are discussed: Abramowitz and Bell 1985; Barkley et al. 1992; Burton, Parker, and Wollner 1991; Carpenter, Heinrichs, and Hanlon 1987; Clarke et al. 1992; Coleman and Kaplan 1990; de-Carufel and Piper 1988; Fairburn et al. 1986; Freemen et al. 1985; Glick et al. 1986; Goldberg and Wool 1985; Hawton et al. 1987; Henggeler 1991; Marmar et al. 1989; Melin and Linton 1988; Resick et al. 1988; Senediak and Spence 1985; Sigrell 1992; Weinstein 1988; Wetzel et al. 1992; Whitlatch, Zarit, and Von Eye 1991.
2. The problem is to discern whether the imperfections in the scales and instruments result in error or bias, or both. To the extent to which the instruments produce measurement error, a study's power to detect differences between groups is reduced. In contrast, if the instrument allows for bias, presumably in the direction of the research hypothesis, then the true differences between groups are exaggerated and statistical significance is illegitimately achieved. The argument is being made throughout the chapters that bias, not simply error, is the problem, and therefore the prudent researcher would be advised to set high significance levels. Yet, in addition to instrument problems, the studies were open to many other sources of bias and error.

   Moreover, many studies accepted the value of an instrument without checking its reliability or using multiple raters. In this way, the false report of an instrument's reliability can encourage studies to exaggerate the effectiveness of an intervention by permitting, as one example, the transmission of researcher expectancy biases. The reported reliabilities of the Beck Depression Inventory, as one example of a widely used scale, seem to be inflated. The conditions under which the reliabilities of the Beck instrument were derived seemed to provide cues for the judges. The inflated reliabilities of the instrument falsely suggest that derived findings result from true instrument measurement and not from imperfections in the instrument that transmit the biases of judges.
3. A large number of other studies of depression are similarly flawed. McLean and Hakstian (1990) also compared a variety of treatments—behavior therapy, pharmacotherapy, psychotherapy, nondirective psychotherapy, and relaxation therapy—and a treatment control, offered in ten weekly sessions, by specialists in each of the therapies. All the groups except the relaxation therapy group, which was the control, suffered attrition rates between 17 percent and 39 percent. While behavior therapy seemed to produce some better scores than the others, there was no consistent pattern of outcomes; the outcome means of all groups were generally indistinguishable. Yet the researchers concluded that ten hours of behavior therapy "had a prophylactic influence over a 2.25-year posttreatment follow-up period for depressed patients, relative to a treatment control condition, whereas other therapies did not."

   Nezu and Perri (1989) reported buoyant results for their experimental subjects who received a short course of "problem-solving therapy." However, their patients were self-selected and only moderately depressed; the study specifically excluded severely distressed patients and those with psychiatric and drug problems. The samples were very small, initially fifteen in each treatment condition and thirteen in the wait-list control, and lost two to attrition in the treatment conditions and two from the wait list. In the end, the lack of representativeness of the research sample, the likelihood of both researcher and subject biases, variations in the skill of the small number of therapists, and the absence of a true nontreatment control completely obscure the value of the findings.

Lewinsohn et al. (1990) employed cognitive-behavioral treatment for depressed adolescents. Hoberman, Lewinsohn, and Tilson (1988) applied the same course to adults. Both reported that the Coping with Depression Course is highly effective. However, the measures in both studies were largely based upon patient self-reports. Samples were small. Blinding procedures were not employed. One study was uncontrolled. Attrition was high. The samples were self-selected and were probably not representative of the population of clinically depressed patients. The largest portion of treatment success could be explained by factors that themselves reduce the severity of the problem of depression (e.g. presence of intimate relationships, less pessimism before treatment, fewer number of previous depressive episodes). In other words, those who needed treatment the least fared the best.

Shapiro et al. (1990) compared cognitive-behavioral therapy with relationship-oriented therapy, provided in either an eight-week or a sixteen-week regimen. This, the Second Sheffield Psychotherapy Project, was designed to correct for the many methodological shortcomings of the First Sheffield Psychotherapy Project. They found substantial clinical improvement. However, all of their outcome assessments were highly reactive to therapist expectations; the assessments were made either by committed therapists or by the patients themselves. "All therapists (were) full-time research clinical psychologists," presumably with large professional and personal stakes in the positive outcomes of their own interventions. No independent or objective assessments were taken. Samples were small; all numbered only twelve.

DeRubeis, Evans, and Hollon (1990) compared the mix of cognitive therapy and pharmacotherapy with pharmacotherapy alone in treating patients with major depressive disorder. Their findings appeared to certify the efficacy of both of their experimental treatments. However, "the difference in depression outcome between [those receiving cognitive therapy together with pharmacotherapy and those receiving pharmacotherapy alone] was small and nonsignificant" (865). Yet, the measures were self-reports and the products of therapist interpretations. Blinding procedures were apparently not employed. Samples were small (thirty-two in both groups). There was no nontreatment control.

Rehm et al. (1981) tested the "contribution of self-evaluation and self-reinforcement modules over and above the self-monitoring module alone" (469). Patients, who were volunteers recruited for the study, received six weekly therapy sessions of a combination of these modules. They found positive results for each of their interventions, but no differences between them. However, they did not employ a nontherapy or placebo control. Their measures were open to both researcher and therapist biases. Interrater reliabilities were not high even on the behavioral measures (.62 to .82), although they "were deemed acceptable." At follow-up, they lost thirty-three out of 104 of their subjects. It is surprising that they considered their samples of approximately thirty to be large. Just two therapists, graduate clinical psychology students, provided all of the therapy. Sample sizes were very small (nine to twelve in treated groups; fifteen on the wait list). While an impressive battery of measures were taken at pre- and posttest, there was no adequate objective check on the possibility that patients in all groups only fulfilled the expectancies of their therapists. Reliability scores among clinician raters were poor, ranging from .60 to .77. It is also uncertain that true blinding was maintained in posttest interviews; evaluators were probably able to pick up cues regarding a patient's assignment to an experimental group or to the wait list.

In similar ways, Bellack, Hersen, and Himmelhoch (1981), Simons et al. (1986), Scogin, Jamison, and Gochneaur (1989), Thompson, Gallagher, and Breckenridge (1987), Jarrett and Nelson (1987), Morris (1987), Rounsaville et al. (1987), Neimeyer and Feixas (1990), and Silverman, Silverman, and Eardley (1984) are also deeply flawed.

Another study, although not including randomized controls, is notable here. The Sokol et al. (1989) study was conducted at the Center for Cognitive Therapy by cognitive therapists, notably A. T. Beck. Not surprisingly, they found that cognitive therapy succeeded in reducing

> panic attacks significantly...to zero by the end of treatment; this improvement in panic and other associated symptoms was maintained at 1-year follow-up... [therefore] cognitive therapy has been shown to provide an alternative to pharmacological treatment of panic disorder. Marked improvement in panic frequency and its maintenance at one year follow-up, along with reductions in depression and general anxiety support this conclusion. (716)

While the authors acknowledged that "the lack of a control group makes efficacy interpretations problematic," they still insisted that "despite these limitations, the current study provides strongly suggestive data regarding the applicability of non-drug treatment to panic disorder" (715). Yet, their sample included only seventeen patients drawn from their own treatment center, many of whom "specifically sought treatment with cognitive therapy" while their measures were largely based upon patient self-report. This study is the more typical research product in psychotherapy because no control group—indeed, no comparison group of any type—was utilized. As a result, their conclusions relative to any treatment are logically baseless.

4. Mattick and Peters (1988) improved on Marchione et al.'s (1987) outcomes, but not on their methods. As in many other studies, Williams, Kinney, and Falbo (1989) do not describe the treatment itself. It is particularly noteworthy in this study because the "therapists were a psychologist and a doctoral student in counseling psychology trained by the psychologist" (438). Klosko et al. (1990) compared chemotherapy with behavior therapy. While their results were significantly better than their placebo control and the wait-list control, the reported results were not significantly better than drug therapy alone and, therefore, the presentation of their conclusions is misleading. Moreover, the behavior group was less debilitated before treatment than the group that only received drug treatment, perhaps accounting in itself for the apparent success of behavior therapy. Schulte et al. (1992) randomized phobic subjects between three therapy conditions. However, a number of problems prevent accepting even their modest conclusions.
5. In another study of posttraumatic stress disorder, Keane, Fairbank, and Caddell (1989) tested the effectiveness of fourteen to sixteen ninety-minute sessions of implosive flooding therapy on a group of Vietnam veterans. It is noteworthy that their major findings were based upon their softest measures and that significant findings, when they occurred, usually took place in pre-posttest therapy measures of the treated group and not between the final levels or degree of improvement achieved by the treated group in comparison with the control. Flooding therapy is an unpleasant experience; patient self-reports may contain inaccura-

cies motivated by their desire to avoid additional therapy. Cooper and Clum (1989) corroborated Keane, Fairbank, and Caddell (1989) with smaller samples (seven in each condition), while repeating all of its methodological flaws.

6. The other contemporary research is generally inferior to Kazdin et al. (1989), while focusing even more tightly on inexpensive interventions. Pisterman, McGrath, and Firestone (1989) employed a delayed treatment control to test the effectiveness of parent-mediated treatment of preschoolers with attention deficit disorder. This may be an instance of the failure of research conducted in a "laboratory" to succeed in the "field." In Kane and Kendall's (1989) experiment, "*four* children diagnosed with overanxious disorder were treated individually with a sixteen to twenty-session, cognitive-behavior treatment that was evaluated using assessments from multiple sources and a multiple-baseline across cases design for the self-reports" (499). They made much of their uncontrolled cases. Manne, Redd, and Jacobsen (1990) "investigated a behavioral intervention incorporating parent coaching, attentional distraction, and positive reinforcement to control child distress during invasive cancer treatment" (565). They tortured their findings to realize their expectations, but while the researchers declared success, the children still hurt.
7. In a weak design, Yohman, Schaeffer, and Parsons (1988) tested a variety of interventions on inpatient alcoholic men and found they were not effective.

   Carroll, Rounsaville, and Gawin (1991) compared relapse prevention psychotherapy with interpersonal psychotherapy in treating cocaine abuse. Against all common expectations, they reported that relapse prevention psychotherapy was significantly more effective than interpersonal psychotherapy with severe substance abusers. However, the findings relied entirely upon patient self-reports, notoriously unreliable when the patients are drug abusers. The patient self-reports were not checked against blood or urine analyses. Furthermore, attrition rates were enormous; 33 percent in the relapse prevention group and 62 percent in the interpersonal psychotherapy group. The study itself pushes against tolerances for self-serving reports. Nevertheless, it was funded by the National Institute on Drug Abuse and conducted at the Yale Medical School.

   Litt et al. (1992) tested the relative effectiveness of two alternative aftercare treatments for alcoholic men, reporting that different types of therapy were successful with different types of alcoholic men. However, they made too much out of their very equivocal findings with relatively small samples. While they did find differences for outcomes that were measured as the amount of time to the first drinking day, all treatment differences evaporated when the criterion was defined as the amount of time to the first *heavy* drinking day (i.e., more than six drinks). In addition, no differences between the treatments were found for psychosocial outcomes—psychiatric severity, social functioning, and employment status. The samples were small and no placebo control was employed. Censoring increased over time with a 23 percent loss of data by the eighteen-month follow-up.

   Kang et al. (1991) evaluated the effectiveness of three different therapies in treating cocaine abusers. "The results of the study indicate that outpatient therapy once a week is ineffective for cocaine use disorder." However, the number of therapy sessions attended was not related to improvement, while the research is beset by methodological problems. In an understated conclusion, referring to Smith, Glass, and Miller (1980), the authors commented that "the finding of no association between number of treatment sessions and improved outcome is at variance with the results of studies that have shown a relationship between amount of treatment received and outcome after treatment of substance abuse disorders."

Sannibale (1989) randomized ninety-six male alcoholics among two brief treatment conditions and a minimal intervention control. Sannibale reported large gains in all of her interventions for alcoholism—approximately half of each group improved. However, the findings are based upon a self-selected group of patients who presented themselves for treatment and upon their self-reports. Randomization produced three groups that differed greatly in important measures of the severity of alcoholism. Most damaging to the findings, gains were largely made by patients with less severe and minimal problems but equivalently among the different groups. Bond et al. (1991) randomized ninety-seven clients with mental illness and substance abuse problems to two different treatment conditions—assertive community treatment and reference groups—and a standard treatment control. Treatment was provided over an eighteen-month period through three community mental health centers. Their "statistical analyses, however, showed few advantages for either treatment program compared to controls."

8. Telch, Agras, and Rossiter (1990) and Pyle et al. (1990), two other randomized studies of treatments for bulimia, were similarly defective.
9. A number of other randomized studies, reporting positive results for a variety of disorders, were also seriously flawed by small samples, researcher biases, subject self-reports, and other problems. Alden (1989) compared three treatments—graduated expose, interpersonal skills training, and intimacy focus—with a nontreatment control in treating avoidant personality disorder (clinical shyness). Piper et al. (1990) studied the impact of one particular pretherapy characteristic—quality of object relations, "defined as a person's tendency to establish certain kinds of relationships with others"—on the outcomes of short-term dynamically oriented individual psychotherapy for psychiatric problems(476). Baggs and Spence (1990) tested the effectiveness of booster sessions in maintaining the gains of assertion training. Flowers and Booraem (1991) compared psychoeducational group therapy with experiential group therapy in treating clients with heterogeneous problems.

4

Recent Tests of the Effectiveness of Family Therapy

Family psychotherapy is advertised as a particularly efficient form of psychotherapy that treats a more complex system—the family—than individual therapy or even group therapy. It is largely based upon the idea that dysfunctional families either create personal problems for their members or fail to adequately satisfy the needs of their members and that under a variety of circumstances the individual is best treated along with his or her family. During recent decades family therapy has focused on divorce and problems with children. Family dissolution has been implicated as the principal causes of violence, crime, and drug and alcohol addiction. Enthusiasts for family therapy claim that evidence has proved its effectiveness beyond question, thereby establishing its utility in addressing serious social problems.

Misleading research that falsely endorses the effectiveness of family therapy has a pernicious effect on social dialectics, depriving distressed families of a just advocacy. Indeed, the problems of contemporary American families may reflect underlying social and economic pressures in the society, particularly the need for two-income households that deprive children of time with their parents. In this case, the failure of family therapy to restore families or to prevent family disintegration would underscore the desirability of more thoroughgoing and proportionately expensive social remedies to relieve the economic distress of families or to buttress their traditional roles: wage supplements and higher minimum wages, demogrants for children, child day care, improved training and educational systems, higher welfare benefits, and so forth. However, all of these remedies, requiring both substantial redistribution of income and government growth, are vastly more expensive than a few hours of family therapy.

Moreover, a strategy of social remedies for family dissolution emphasizes an ideology that locates the major causes and, consequently, the responsibility to alleviate family distress in the structure of the society and not in the failings of individuals. In this sense, imperfections in the social order that threaten family integrity justify the provision of supplemental services and other social reforms. In contrast, family therapy, locating the source of family distress in the pathological behaviors of family members, tacitly places the onus on the families themselves to make appropriate adaptations to the culture.

By either endorsing or discrediting family therapy, each outcome study in the field enters the social dispute over claims to scarce resources. Therefore, whatever its scholarly merits, each study is a factional statement that supports particular political and economic contestants.

Family therapy has been prescribed for a broad range of conditions: anxiety, personality disorders, drug and alcohol addiction, impulse control, and adjustment problems. Across the range of disorders, family therapy is predicated upon a few central assumptions. First, the family is an operational system and, therefore, the behavior of the family system "is best understood as a product of its organizational characteristics" (*Treatments of Psychiatric Disorders,* hereafter referred to as TPD 1989, 2567). In this way, the dysfunctional behavior of a family member is best interpreted as an adaptation to the dysfunctions of the family itself. Consequently, family functioning affects the emergence of symptoms as well as their intensity. Even when the disease has a biological grounding (e.g. organic aggressive syndrome and schizophrenia) family psychotherapy may still provide a useful palliative as a social treatment that minimizes the family's role in exacerbating symptoms.

Secondly, the family's role in creating stress among its members is frequently identified as the vehicle that initiates and sustains symptoms. Family psychotherapy, therefore, focuses on minimizing the family's role in creating stress with the consequence that a variety of problems caused by stress (e.g. anxiety and personal maladjustment) are amenable to actual cure.

> Family stress theory, as underscored by the Typology Model of Family Adjustment and Adaptation, emphasizes the importance of established patterns or typologies of family functioning which, if understood, can serve well the therapist, crisis manager, and educator. Helping families to move from being a Fragile family unit...to be Resilient...or moving the family from Intentional...to being a Rhythmic

> family unit...are legitimate and measurable objectives. Current research...provide us with initial evidence that these family types—Resilient, Rhythmic, and Regenerative—may be at the hub of family functioning. (McCubbin and McCubbin, 39)

Finally, the practice of family psychotherapy identifies the social environment in which the individual resides—not just a patient's intrapsychic experience—as the telling factor that influences personal behavior, even when the initial cause of the problem is biological. However, the field defines family life as the critical social environment that must be repaired in order to restore people to proper functioning. In short, the effectiveness of family psychotherapy is predicated upon the assumptions that individual deviance can be corrected by restoring appropriate family functioning, and that this restoration is possible through family psychotherapy.

There are a variety of therapeutic approaches to treat families. They break down roughly along the same lines as individual psychotherapy: cognitive (also called cognitive-behavioral) approaches based upon some form of rational induction, and behavioral approaches that attempt to directly manipulate reinforcements.

In a manner similar to the previous review of individual and group therapy, the best of the research evidence for the effectiveness of family therapy from 1980 through 1992 was identified through reviews of the secondary literature and through reviews of the journals themselves.[1]

The Outcome Research

The goals of the outcome studies were not modest. Each study set out to test the value of specific techniques of family therapy in achieving important social goals: preservation and improvement of marriage, reduction in psychotic behavior, and the adjustment of delinquent and problem children. The researchers justified their studies on the basis of their theoretical and practical value. All of the outcome studies evaluated relatively inexpensive, short-term treatments.

Research subjects were usually selected from among those who were seeking treatment from an agency or those who were already in therapy. No study defined a population at risk then established a recruitment procedure.

The typical sample was under twenty; many were under ten. In no case did a sample contain more than 100 subjects. While procedures to test for statistical significance implicitly adjust for the size of samples, smaller samples are more vulnerable to researcher and sampling biases. It is far more difficult to influence thousands than it is to influence just a few. Frequently study participants were selected subsequent to an interview in which both objective criteria (e.g., drug free, living with spouse) and subjective criteria (e.g., sincerity about therapy) were applied.

The therapists who delivered the treatments were frequently psychologists and psychiatrists. However, many of the therapists were trained nurses, social workers, and graduate and undergraduate students. The use of relatively inexpensive therapists increased the efficiency of already inexpensive interventions.

The therapists and the researchers were frequently the same people, although some studies trained their own therapists, but usually by the researchers themselves. The therapists who were graduate and undergraduate students frequently were studying under the researchers and their faculty colleagues. No study recruited independent therapists or independent researchers in an attempt to study the live practice situation in the field. Many studies made efforts to assure treatment integrity by providing the therapists with consistent instructions and manuals and by monitoring their sessions with patients through audio- and videotaping.

Typically the measures of subject performance were applied before therapy, just after therapy and, in a number of studies, at a variety of follow-up intervals, but usually less than one year. One three-year and one four-year follow-up were reported.

This generation of outcome research in family therapy typically employed a controlled design in which an initial pool of research subjects were randomly assigned to experimental conditions, placebo controls, or, more commonly, wait-list controls. Particularly in this regard, current research in the field is superior to earlier cohorts of studies that were usually uncontrolled. However, most often the control group was a standard treatment or an alternative treatment. Moreover, neither the researchers nor the therapists were usually blind to the subjects' assignment. The subjects and their families were also frequently aware of whether they were experimental subjects or controls.

It is often impossible to blind the person delivering the treatment to a patients' status. It is, however, often possible to blind the raters—those assessing outcomes—to the status of the subjects who they are rating.

Yet, even in the many instances in which it was possible, not one study employed specific blinding procedures.

Many researchers may have consciously attempted to minimize the impact of their own expectations in determining study outcomes by employing systematic, "objective" assessment tools. However, these tools frequently required subjective ratings to be applied by the therapists, the researchers, or a research staff. Often these measures depended upon the self-report of patients or their families. The reliability of many of the scales was not firmly established in prior research. A few of the studies employed truly objective measures (e.g., urinalysis for drug use, body weight as a sign of recovery from anorexia) but most did not. Few studies checked the reliability of their measurement instruments or employed multiple raters. Rather, they inaccurately assumed, sometimes on the basis of faulty reports of reliability studies that appeared in the literature, that their measures were reliable. This assumption greatly improved the chance of demonstrating that their experimental interventions were superior to their controls, especially when the instruments were porous enough to transmit raters' biases.

The Treatments and their Outcomes

Schizophrenia, Depression, Anorexia Nervosa, Obsessive-Compulsive Disorder

Short-term family therapy—customarily provided in less than a few months of weekly sessions—is apparently an effective treatment for persisting psychiatric disorders (Hafner et al. 1983), schizophrenia (Leff, Kuipers, Berkowitz, et al. 1982; Falloon 1982), depression (O'Leary and Beach 1990; Beach and O'Leary 1986), obsessive compulsive patients (Emmelkamp and DeLange 1983), and anorexia nervosa and bulimia nervosa (Russell et al. 1987).

However, in all of these studies samples were consistently small. Nontreatment controls were not routinely employed. Many measures were subjective. Researchers were frequently therapists and raters. Long-term follow-ups were not conducted.

Moreover, most of these studies employed combinations of family psychotherapy and social supports as their experimental interventions. It is particularly noteworthy that the absence of appropriate controls created a pointed theoretical problem even if the outcomes of the studies had been credible. The studies could not distinguish between the need for sustained social supports and the need for their short-term family psychotherapy interventions. This is of major importance in estimating the costs for successful long-term treatment of psychiatric patients, particularly schizophrenics. It is probable that relapse—measured as rehospitalization—will increase as the *social* supports of the tested interventions (surveillance of the patients' needs, particularly medication; supervision of relatives; provision of a secure, nonabusive environment; and so forth) are removed. Moreover, even when moderately successful, none of the studies can identify the critical elements of treatment that produced the changes.

This confusion in cause is made against the backdrop of a declining public commitment to fulfill the promise to deinstitutionalize chronic mental health patients. The essence of community psychiatry and the community mental health movement lay in the case management of severely impaired psychotics, usually schizophrenics, and the availability of a range of social supports that allowed them to adapt to a community setting. However, these services cost *more* than hospitalization (Stein and Test 1980) and consequently, over the past fifteen years, an increasingly unsympathetic society has retrenched its commitment to community care.

The suggestion that family therapy is in some way an important ingredient in community care or that it compensates for thin social supports endorses the public policy strategies of a declining welfare state. The faulty research that has produced the perception that family therapy is an important ingredient in the treatment of severely ill patients hides their true needs from the policy debate. Not coincidentally, it supplants social concern with medical attention, advancing the authority of the physician over a problem that may only respond to the provision of humane and homelike environments in the least restrictive setting. However, the routine provision of those services greatly exceed the cost of a few hours of family therapy. In this light, the imprecision of the research serves politically conservative ends by obscuring the determinants of effective treatment.

Marital Therapy for Marital Problems

Family psychotherapy has expended an immense amount of attention on marital problems. The effectiveness of marital psychotherapy in either improving marriage or avoiding divorce has been tested by a large number of researchers.[2] Typically, treatments involved fewer than twenty sessions; rarely was a patient or couple seen for more than fifty sessions. The sessions usually lasted approximately one and one half hours and involved discussions between the married couple and a trained therapist. A few samples of the best research are discussed below.

Because behavioral marital therapy assumes that "disturbed marital interaction... [results] from low rates of positive reinforcement exchanged by couples, a major treatment strategy is to increase positive control while decreasing the rate of aversive control" (Nichols and Schwartz 1991, 339). Following formal learning theory, the behavioral marital therapist prescribes a series of interactions between spouses to increase their positive reinforcing behavior and to decrease their negative interactions. The therapy sessions are used to assess and to treat targeted behaviors:

> Several relationship skills are evaluated, including the ability to discuss relationship problems, current reinforcement value for one another, skill in pinpointing relevant reinforcers in the relationship, competencies in sex, childrearing, financial management, distribution of roles, and decision-making. Interviews are used to specify and elaborate target behaviors, first revealed on the structured assessment devices. (Nichols and Schwartz 1991, 339)

O'Farrell, Cutter, and Floyd (1985) reported that behavioral marital therapy "brought alcoholics with serious marital and drinking problems into the range of nondistressed marital couples" (163). Moreover, they noted that "alcoholics in all three groups (this included the control) showed very substantial short-term improvements in their drinking." But they can not discount alternative possibilities that these improvements occurred as a result of a placebo effect, as the result of seeking treatment itself, or as a result of the special motivation of the study's highly selective group of patients that may distinguish them from the underlying population of families with alcoholics. All of their samples numbered only between nine and twelve. Moreover, the improvements occurred on the most subjective outcome measures, those depending upon patient report. Outcomes were least significant where some objectivity was introduced into the evaluations.

Baucom and Lester (1986) evaluated cognitive restructuring in behavioral marital therapy. Cognitive restructuring seeks to change belief systems, assuming that more congruent attitudes between spouses will reduce their problems. It requires patients to monitor their thoughts:

> A major part of the therapy then consists of getting patients to learn how to evaluate their thoughts, specifically to become alert to those that are irrational and inappropriate. It has been discovered that a variety of cognitive distortions are commonly held to be truths. For example, that "there is invariably a right, precise, and perfect solution to human problems and that it is catastrophic if the correct solution is not found." (TPD 1989, 2542)

Cognitive restructuring as an adjunct to behavioral marital therapy was administered to distressed couples in twelve weekly conjoint sessions each lasting 1.5 hours. Baucom and Lester (1986) concluded that,

> at posttest and follow-up, approximately half of the persons receiving treatment moved into the nondistressed range of marital adjustment. Recently, Follette, Jacobson, Wood, Katt and Follette (1984) presented almost identical improvement rates for all couples receiving BMT.... More specifically Follette's improvement rates were no more than 2 percent different from our overall improvement rates at either posttest or 6-month follow-up. Thus, using the Dyadic Adjustment Scale as a criterion, some confidence can be placed in the expectation that approximately half of the spouses treated with BMT will be no longer significantly distressed by the end of therapy.

However, by the six-month follow-up many of the gains had been lost while the follow-up data were based upon *fewer than 25 percent* of the patients. Their carefully phrased conclusion was based upon an analysis of research groups that contained fewer than nine couples each. Out of twenty analytic cells, three were empty, and nine contained only one subject. The Dyadic Adjustment Scale was self-reported by the patients. Moreover,

> the therapists were two clinical psychologists who were the principal investigators of the study. The first investigator had 8 years of experience and the second investigator 5 years conducting BMT when the investigations began.... [T]his investigation provided an opportunity to examine the effectiveness of more experienced therapists. (Baucom and Lester 1986, 399)

Experienced therapists or compromised researchers? The therapists gathered the pretest and posttest data. Therefore the couples may have attempted to please the therapists; similar demand characteristics across therapy conditions could actually contribute to a lack of significant differences between the two active therapy conditions. Presumably the couples' desire to please the therapists also vitiated the differences between the controls and the experimental couples.

Nichols and Schwartz (1991), in their prominent textbook of family therapy, make a curious observation about behavioral marital therapy: "[M]ost forms of psychotherapy begin as art and move toward science; behavioral marriage therapy did the reverse, beginning as science and moving toward art" (338). Yet art in this context, proffered as an imaginative strength of the field when perhaps it should be seen as an evasion of rational accountability, employs largely verbal tools, even exhortations of the therapist to "accentuate the positive" (Nichols and Schwartz 1991, 339). Aside from ignoring the deeper antecedents of current behaviors, behavioral marital therapy treatments, especially when abetted with cognitive restructuring, appear similar to cognitive interventions while both apparently assume that the therapeutic milieu is sufficient to correct marital problems. Except for assigned homework, treatment is confined to the therapist's office and therefore, the terrain of a couple's problems seem simply to be located in their interactions, divorced from the broader social context. This limitation is rarely addressed by researchers directly; it would severely threaten psychotherapy as a remedy for social problems.

Snyder and Wills (1989) administered twenty-five sessions of either behavioral or insight-oriented therapy. In this case, behavior marital therapy involved "communication skills, problem-solving skills, relationship enhancement, and contingency contracting—all of which emphasized immediate changes in the couples interactions and the development of relationship competency" (41). Insight-oriented therapy seeks to bring about change in marriage through the couple's understanding of the problems in their interactions. It underplays the reinforcing role of interactions in favor of the possibility that rational understanding is sufficient to induce change.

Snyder and Wills (1989) "present evidence for both the significance and the general equivalence of behavioral and insight-oriented marital therapies in producing positive changes in interspousal and intrapersonal functioning." However, the outcome data were self-reported by patients. Samples contained fewer than thirty subjects. The therapists were all trained by one of the researchers.

In contrast to Snyder and Wills (1989), Snyder, Wills, and Grady-Fletcher's (1991) four-year follow-up reported that "significant differences in marital status and rates of deterioration between couples receiving behavioral versus insight-oriented marital therapies were unexpected," especially since they did not appear during the follow-up period. Thirty-eight percent of couples in the behavioral group (but only three percent of the insight group) had divorced by the follow-up. Some therapists do not consider divorce to be a negative outcome of marital therapy even while it constitutes "deterioration among couples."

Nonetheless, divorce is an objective measure. Yet, despite these differences in divorce rates, "there were no differences across treatment conditions in responses to other questionnaire items regarding marital or other problems since termination" (Snyder, Wills, and Grady-Fletcher 1991, 140). However, the researchers should have been concerned that self-reported data, subjectively assessing the patients's conditions, did not seem to be good predictors of important behavioral events, (e.g., divorce). These contradictory findings reinforce skepticism toward the value of patient self-reports, especially when the interactions among researchers, therapists, and patients may strongly influence the patient's judgments.

Family therapists have argued for the necessity of treating both spouses. Szapocznik et al. (1983) entered the debate over conjoint versus one-person family therapy through a study of brief strategic family therapy lasting twelve sessions.

> Like behaviorists, strategic therapists focus on behavior, and are not concerned with insight. However, they differ from behaviorists in one important respect—behaviorists rely on the power of rational instruction; strategic therapists eschew understanding altogether. They do not believe in insight, and they do not believe in teaching; instead they believe that the way to change behavior is through manipulation. They box stuck families into a corner, from which the only way out is to become unstuck. (Nichols and Schwartz 1991, 542)

Szapocznik et al. (1983) reported that conjoint and one-person brief strategic family therapy were both effective *in spite of the fact that they did not outperform the recreational control group*. Yet, the huge amount of differential attrition (almost 50 percent by the follow-up assessment) vitiates any finding. Nonetheless, Szapocznik et al. (1983) attempted to convert the higher attrition in the control group into a virtue by stating that the ability to hold patients is an important therapeutic outcome.

They interpreted the decline in family functioning that followed one-person family therapy as a sign of successful therapy. "One of the central tenets of family systems theory... is that the child, the identified patient, is serving an active role in holding the family together by helping the family avoid other problems" (Szapocznik et al. 1983, 576). As successful therapy with the young boys began to deprive their families of a scapegoat, their families began to disintegrate, leading the authors to claim "that this is the first time that such a basic assumption of family systems theory has been demonstrated quantitatively" (Szapocznik et al. 1983, 576). In contrast, if the reverse had occurred, that is, if the families did not disintegrate, then the researchers could also have claimed success. Thus, through the logic of *ex post facto* analysis, the research was protected from failure. This being the case, there was no need to conduct the research in the first place. The existence of criteria to distinguish between experimental failure and success is a necessary hallmark of true research.

The logic of their own experimental design should have driven the authors to conclude that neither of their experimental conditions was more effective than their control. Instead, they insisted in the face of their own disconfirming evidence and weak methodology that "there are several important findings in this study" (Szapocznik et al. 1983, 575).

Couples' communication has been a popular form of marital psychotherapy. It assumes that improper communication is the root cause of marital distress. The therapist acts as a process leader, relating democratically to the family members, with little concern for family structure even including the parents' position of authority.

> The goal of the communications therapist is, like that of the behavior therapist, to interdict behaviors that stimulated and reinforced symptoms.... If behavior is communication, then the way to change behavior is to change communication. According to the communications theorists, all events and actions have communicative properties: Symptoms can be considered as covert messages, commenting upon relationships. (Nichols and Schwartz 1991, 203)

Girodo, Stein, and Dotzenroth (1980) tested the effectiveness of the Minnesota Couples Communication Program on "moderately distressed couples." The therapy consisted of five weekly training sessions. According to the architects of the Minnesota Couples Communication Program,

> each session builds on the experience of previous exercises, simulations, discussions and reading of *Alive and Aware: Improving the Communication in Relationships*. The book supplements the lectures and provides a number of exercises to help couples practice at home and transfer their learning to their relationship outside the group context. Each of the...sessions focuses on one framework. Along with the framework, a set of skills is presented and practices which links in with specific parts of the framework. The four frameworks are as follows [Awareness Wheel, Shared Meaning Process, Communications Styles, and I Count/I Count You]. (Miller, Nunnally, and Wackman 1976, 29)

Girodo, Stein, and Dotzenroth (1980) obtained mixed results for their study of communication therapy for couples who "at least had thought of divorce but had not gone as far as seeking legal counsel" (64). However, only twenty-four couples were randomized to three treatment groups and a control. The measures were self-reports. Joanning (1982) treated couples who had requested counseling from a university counseling service. They received "the standard four week Couple Communication Agenda and engaged in homework activities outlined in the Couple Workbook" (465). Joanning discovered across-the-board improvements for couples who were treated in the communication program. However, the gains did not persist at a five-month follow-up. Only seventeen couples were treated. Measures were self-reported. No control was employed.

Brock and Joanning (1983) compared two types of communication skills training programs—relationship enhancement and a standard couples communication approach. Therapy time in each condition totaled twenty hours with trained leaders. Brock and Joanning (1983) found that the Relationship Enhancement Program was superior to the Minnesota Couples Communication Program. Yet, each sample contained only twenty-six couples. The nonrandom control contained only eight. Outcome data were collected via subject self-reports and evaluations by independent raters of videotaped interactions. The differences between the groups were small, although statistically significant, and of questionable clinical or theoretical value.

Indeed, the couples communication interventions are so superficial that it seems questionable whether they are capable of having any impact at all on severe marital problems. Moreover, the subjects may not have been distressed to begin with. Participants were self-selected and many may have attended these programs recreationally, as other couples attend church meetings, take up bridge, or go on vacations to exotic locations. The marital family therapy literature is consistently silent on the social causation of family distress as well as the difficulty of treating families in isolation from their social environment. Yet most family distress, perhaps frequently expressed as poor communication, may reflect the inability of many American families to cope with new social and economic pressures—notably the necessity for two-earner families. The situation is even more difficult for single heads of families:

> Exactly what is it about the changing American family that is a problem?.... [I]t is that the marriage bond is steadily weakening. Children are spending less time with

> their parents for many reasons, but especially due to the growing absence of their fathers. Across society, children's needs are often placed behind those of adults. In short, the child-centered, two parent family shows growing signs of disintegration, reflected most clearly in the continued high rate of divorce and the steady growth in the number of unwed parents. (Popenoe 1993, A48)

It is both a professional conceit and a polemical convenience of the socially efficient myth that family therapy is in any way an equivalent substitute for adequate incomes, attentive parents, child day care, safe communities, effective schools, and a fair job market.

Family Therapy with Children

Szapocznik et al. (1989) compared structural family therapy and psychodynamic child therapy with a recreational control in the treatment of emotional and behavioral problems among Hispanic boys. All of the treatments "spanned a maximum of a 6-month period with a minimum of 12 and a maximum of 24 contact hours" by a single therapist (572). Psychodynamic child psychotherapy, rooted in Freudian psychoanalysis, employs techniques of depth psychology that attempt to discover and interpret unconscious impulses and the individual's defenses against them. Consequently, the goal of the psychodynamic treatment condition in Szapocznik et al. (1989) was to eliminate unconscious restrictions to appropriate family functioning.

> In this widely used, nondirective approach, the child was seen in a playroom situation, and the mother was seen briefly as an adjunctive aid. Expression of feelings, limit setting transference interpretations, and insight as a mechanism for change were emphasized. (Szapocznik et al., 572)

In contrast, structural family therapy, promoted by Salvador Minuchin, is a directive approach. Family structures are repeated, organized patterns of behavior through which a family interacts. The therapist attempts to interrupt dysfunctional patterns of behavior and introduce more appropriate structures by utilizing a variety of techniques.

> Structural family therapists believe that problems are maintained by dysfunctional family structures. Therefore therapy is directed at altering family structure so that the family can solve its problems.... The structural family therapist joins the family system in order to help its members change their structure. By altering boundaries and realigning subsystems, the therapist changes the behavior and experience of each of the family members. (Nichols and Schwartz 1991, 460)

Szapocznik et al. (1989) reported that "the two treatment conditions were essentially equivalent in reducing behavioral and emotional problems based on parent reports and self-reports, relatively equivalent in improving psychodynamic ratings of child functioning and significantly different in protecting family integrity in the long term" (576). Yet, the three treatment conditions "did not differ significantly among themselves" (575). However, the improvements of the recreational control were not subtracted from the treatment group improvements to derive a true measure of effects. This procedure would have reduced already low, albeit significant effects to insubstantial levels especially in light of the study's other methodological problems. Attrition was much higher in the control group than in the experimental group. Samples were small and highly selective. Many of the measures of outcomes were not objective. Therapists, and frequently raters, were aware of the group assignment of subjects. By falsely insisting upon the benefits of family psychotherapy, Szapocznik et al. (1989) perversely deny their subjects—in this case, members of a deprived minority—of a just advocacy. For, if the minimal interventions of family psychotherapy cannot engineer appropriate adjustment, then more intense interventions—perhaps dealing directly with the inadequacies of schools, communities, and subcultures themselves—become live policy options. Ironically, the failure of the study's interventions, reflecting the inadequacies of the psychotherapy generally, are tributes to Minuchin's insistence that the therapist needs to look beyond the family itself in order to address many of its problems (Elizur and Minuchin 1989).

The Szapocznik findings minimize the degree to which family distress reflects the institutionalized social inequalities of the broader culture. The study, failing as credible clinical science, is best interpreted as a factional justification of "culturally sensitive" professional interventions at the expense of more thoroughgoing social interventions.

Manne, Redd, and Jacobsen (1990) "investigated a behavioral intervention incorporating parent coaching, attentional distraction, and positive reinforcement to control child distress during invasive cancer treatment" (565). "Intervention consisted of instruction in attentional distraction, paced breathing and positive reinforcement... [it] was conducted in a private area by a clinical psychologist for approximately 10 minutes before" the first trial (566).

However, Manne, Redd, and Jacobsen (1990) tortured their findings to realize their expectations, concluding that

> behavioral intervention incorporating parent coaching, attentional distraction, and positive reinforcement produced marked reductions in children's behavioral distress, parents' anxiety, and parents' ratings of child pain. However, the intervention did not influence children's perceptions of their own pain or nurses' ratings of child pain and distress. (570)

In other words, the researchers declared success, but the children still hurt. The researchers then attempted to invalidate the nurse's reports. "[O]ne possible explanation is that the nurse's rating was influenced more by her own level of anxiety than by the child's anxiety" (571). They also attempted to reinterpret the children's report. But they did not consider the possibility that their own needs to report success distorted the design and interpretation of their study and they ignore the more direct implication of their findings that their intervention was a failure.

Lieberman, Weston, and Pawl (1991) tested the value of attachment theory psychotherapy as a preventive intervention "to promote secure attachment" between immigrant Mexican mothers and their infants in the second year of life:

> [Attachment theory] intends to provide the mother with a corrective attachment experience. The intervenor spoke for the mother's affective experience, addressing the legitimacy of her longings for protection and safety both when she was a child and currently as an adult, and enabling her to explore unsettling feelings of anger and ambivalence toward others (including the child and the intervenor).... When feasible, the intervenor also tried to provide concrete elements of protection by helping to secure needed goods and services. (Lieberman, Weston, and Pawl, 1991, 202)

The authors "surmised that the infants would be at risk for anxious attachment because their mothers might be relatively emotionally unavailable due to their circumstances" (i.e., low socioeconomic status and the high incidence of depression, anxiety, and unemployment among recent Mexican immigrants). However, the mothers who were recruited from pediatric clinics "showed no flagrant psychological disorders" (200). Mother-infant dyads were first classified as secure or anxious; the secure group served as one control and the anxious dyads were then randomized to either a treatment group or a nontreatment control. Treatment was conducted over one year.

> The format was unstructured weekly sessions with mother and baby.... Mothers received $15.00 and transportation costs at the time of each [therapy] visit.... The

> intervenors sought to alleviate the mothers' psychological conflicts about their children and to provide developmental information that was clinically timed and tailored to the child's temperament and individual style.... In attachment theory language, this intervention approach intends to provide the mother with a corrective attachment experience. (202)

Outcomes were measured at the end of the one-year therapy and one year later. Lieberman, Weston, and Pawl (1991) reported findings that "suggest that the intervention was effective in enhancing maternal empathy and interaction with the child; decreasing toddler avoidance, resistance, and anger; and increasing goal-corrected partnership" (206). However, they made too much of their findings, which were marginally significant and inconsistent. In addition, the groups were small and attrition in the experimental procedure exceeded 20 percent. Presumably, the attrition masked therapeutic failures that were not accounted for in the measured outcomes.

Moreover, there were large initial differences between the experimental group and the nontreatment control. Although all of these differences, except for one, were not statistically significant, they were frequently large enough and important enough to raise serious questions about whether the outcomes were due to the intervention or to natural and selective reductions in these group differences. Fewer of the children in the experimental group than in the control group were in day care and more of them were first born. Moreover, the one statistically significant difference occurred in employment. Fully 54 percent of experimental group families were unemployed, while only 15 percent of the anxious control group were unemployed. The observed reduction of anxiety-related behaviors in the experimental group may have been due to their simple acculturation—finding day care, employment, and information about childrearing—that was not related to the therapeutic intervention but was probably related to being in the United States for a few years. In this light, the nontreatment control should have been a placebo control, perhaps one that provided simple information to the immigrant mothers in contrast to the therapy condition that also applied the rare professional skills of attachment theory therapy.

Furthermore, the outcome observations by trained raters may have been open to a variety of biases since blinding may have been frequently breached. It is also quite possible that therapists transmitted their expectancies to their patients by encouraging behaviors that were particularly germane to the evaluation procedure, conducted during a final session in which patient outcomes were observed. In addition, these clinical behaviors themselves may not have been pertinent to the relationship between mothers and children, but only a reflection of therapist-induced mimicking. Finally, interrater reliabilities were frequently modest while the concurrent validity correlations of their "empathic responsiveness scale" (.43 and .38) were very poor.

However, none of these serious threats to the value of the study deterred the authors from announcing important insights on the basis of their research:

> Maternal involvement in the therapeutic process appears as a key variable in fostering adaptive change.... The findings suggest that assessing the mother's use of intervention should become an integral part of intervention research in infant mental health. (Lieberman, Weston, and Pawl 1991)

The findings provided little support for any of these notions or for the value of attachment therapy itself. The study did not demonstrate that important problems among relatively well adjusted immigrant families were averted by attachment therapy. Rather the research results suggested that superficial family interventions—1.5 hours of weekly home visits over a year—have little impact, if any at all, on mother-child relations.

Miscellaneous

Family therapy is apparently a highly effective remedy for agoraphobia. Barlow, O'Brien, and Last (1984) treated agoraphobics in

> twelve weekly, 60- to 90- minute group discussion sessions, conducted according to a detailed protocol.... [T]he treatment could best be characterized as a self-initiated, graduated-exposure treatment combined with instruction on panic management procedures, as well as cognitive therapy that included the use of coping self-statements, paradoxical intention and similar methods designed to prevent cognitive avoidance of fear. Couples in the spouse group were also encouraged to communicate more effectively during periods of anxiety or panic, and during treatment sessions they negotiated strategies for handling "anxiety" that were acceptable to both partners. (47)

Barlow, O'Brien, and Last (1984) found that

> including husbands directly in the treatment of agoraphobic women provided a substantial clinical advantage...in that 12 out of 14 clients responded to treatment. Women treated without their husbands did not do as well. (52)

The two treatment groups contained only fifteen and fourteen subjects, respectively. No nontreatment control was employed. Ratings were subjective, made by therapists and patients. No follow-up measures were taken. The criteria for successful treatment—20 percent improvement in at least three of the five measures—opened the door to rater bias. However, the flaws in this research were typical of the agoraphobia family treatment research (Cobb et al. 1984; Bland and Hallam 1981; Emmelkamp 1980). In a nutshell, the effectiveness of family psychotherapy in treating agoraphobia still needs to be demonstrated.

Adams, Piercey, and Jurich (1991) compared the effectiveness of three different family therapy treatments. Sixty families, half of whom had problems with their children, were randomly assigned. The first experimental group was given a "formula task" at the end of their first session; the second session was conducted "using a 'solution focused' orientation." This group received an average of 8.85 sessions.

The second group was also given a "formula task" at the end of the their first session; however, the second session did not provide a "solution focused" orientation, while the remainder of their therapy, averaging 8.9 sessions, was conducted largely through a structural-strategic orientation.

The control treatment group received a "problem focused task" at the end of their initial session: "Between now and the next time we meet, we would like you to observe, so that you can describe to us next time, the problems(s) occurring in your (pick one: family, life, marriage, relationship)." Families in the control received an average of 11.5 sessions.

Nichols and Schwartz (1991) place solution-focused therapy at the cutting edge of family psychotherapy. Solution-focused therapists deny that patients are resistant to treatment; when clients do not follow therapeutic advice they are really attempting to teach therapists the best way to help them. Therapists focus on solutions, spending little energy to explore the source of problems.

> Solution-focused therapists borrow from constructivists the idea that there is no true reality, so therapists shouldn't impose what they think is normal on clients. Instead, therapy should concern itself only with the complaints that clients present. Thus...the goals of solution-focused therapists are to resolve the presenting complaints by helping a client do or think something different so as to become more satisfied with his or her life. (Nichols and Schwartz 1991, 483)

Formula tasks are assignments given to patients that stimulate them to search for solutions. These formula tasks seem to work with many patients regardless of their problems. Much of the efforts of solution-focused therapists are invested in searches for effective formula tasks.

Adams, Piercey, and Jurich (1991) found that the "formula first session task" was an effective intervention in the "initial stages of treatment for gaining family compliance, increasing the clarity of treatment goals, and initiating improvement in the presenting problem." However, the ratings depended upon therapist evaluations of the subjects' performance. Although these ratings were checked against the evaluations of two trained "independent observers," the observers were probably neither neutral nor blind to the patients' status. The observers were apparently graduate students in marital and family therapy while they probably picked up cues to the patients' stature from conversations in the taped interviews that they reviewed. Moreover, it is unlikely that the fifteen participating therapists were unaware of the researchers' preferences since they had been given special training in solution-focused therapy (the key experimental variable) as a part of the experiment. Still, the initial ratings of subject improvement by both the therapists and the observers "showed a constricted range" falling largely in two categories, "about the same" and "somewhat better." Therefore, the researchers judged that this variable was "unacceptable for a variance analysis and the Chi-square statistic was adopted to assess differences in the distribution scores on the variable across treatment conditions." It is also highly unlikely that the "independent" raters, who were graduate students in the authors' programs, were any more neutral than the therapists themselves.

Yet, more troubling than a convenient analysis of biased evaluations, even the statistically significant differences between groups were small while the authors failed to establish the relevance of their findings. Indeed, their research, only measuring the process of therapy, failed to assess the actual behavioral outcomes of therapy on the presenting problems. It would be wonderful support for the idea of efficient clinical solutions if important progress could be made against serious personal problems in under ten hours of therapy. However, the researchers failed to establish the gravity of their subjects' problems; no independent or clinical assessment was made of their presenting conditions. The subjects were self-referred to family counseling centers and all of the outcome measures were geared to the subjects' own definitions of their family problems. Moreover, neither the researchers nor the field has credibly established the strategic value of goal clarity, optimism, or compliance in attaining the goals of family psychotherapy. In this regard, the study's positive findings relative to two of these three instrumental variables could also be attributed to bias as well as to the ritualized adaptations of patients to the therapeutic milieu.

Family psychotherapists, especially at the cutting edge, intensely compete for the reputation of success. Their insights are treated reverentially. The shortcomings of Adams, Piercey, and Jurich (1991) epitomize the customary refusal of the field's research to withstand practitioners' demands for findings that corroborate their wisdom and endorse their private practices, consultantships, and training institutes. The practice of family psychotherapy can be quite lucrative. Prominent therapists, especially those with emergent ideas that capture either popular enthusiasms or the field's attentions, own private clinics and practices, provide workshops and seminars for practitioners, affiliate with training institutes, sell books, and pursue consultantships.

Conclusions: The Effectiveness of Family Therapy

Family therapy raises common sense to the level of professional, even medical treatment, but unfortunately without any clinical evidence of effectiveness. The field has produced a defiant literature lacking insight and mired in the aphoristic value of courtesy and concern, especially in marriage: it is good to be good. The range of tested family interventions—psychodynamic therapy, structural therapy, cognitive restructuring, communications therapy, Minnesota Couples Communication Therapy, communication skills training, behavioral marital therapy, insight oriented therapy, relationship enhancement, emotionally focused therapy, brief strategic therapy, multisystem therapy, attachment theory therapy, and others—seem to involve little more than moral preaching. They seem to be largely indistinguishable; their tenets, especially in the outcome literature, are rarely defined in a way that allows specific theoretical ideas to be tested; they are customarily presented in a polemical manner and in an environment that compels acceptance and belief more than rational scrutiny. Moreover, family psychotherapy in all of its different forms seems to be largely responsive to the imperatives of the culture for symbols of family solidarity that transmit a moral orthodoxy. Beleaguered families, not their imperfect environments, are the focus of treatment and the literature has flatly refused to test the ability of psychotherapeutic treatment to compensate for neurotic factors outside of the family.

Yet, precisely because it ignores the social context of family dysfunction, family therapy may be an impossible strategy. Indeed, family therapy remains live in the public imagination in part because the field refuses to conduct true tests of its effectiveness and in part because the political constituency for alternative remedies remains too weak to insist upon objective evaluations.

The contemporary membership in the critical tradition of family therapy is very sparse: Bagarozzi and Rauen (1981), Masten (1979), possibly Wells and Dezen (1978), and perhaps a few others. Typically, the summary reviews of family therapy, even those that tolerated criticism of the field's effectiveness, failed to follow the logic of their own data and the implications of their own comments. They insisted that family therapy is a safe and effective treatment despite their many conscious criticisms of its outcome studies: flawed data, inadequate methodologies, inappropriate analyses, inadequate and nonrepresentative samples, and a variety of biases. Moreover, the selection biases of the field routinely produce research subjects that are far less debilitated than the underlying problem population. As a result, the report of cure is frequently very misleading.

On simple methodological grounds the outcomes of family therapy are indeterminate. Yet the critical tradition in the field has exercised little restraint on the claims of family practitioners, failing to encourage the field's community of scholars to produce credible research. The critical tradition has apparently had little impact on political or social preferences that ignore the experimental, unsubstantiated, indeterminate nature of the practice of family therapy.

The field's factitious studies and their obviously self-protective presentation begin to suggest that family therapy may actually be ineffective and perhaps even harmful, and not just indeterminate. Placebo effects may account for most of the reported positive outcomes while the tyranny of grouped data force the conclusion that at least some deterioration takes place. Furthermore, the very reactive measures that are usually taken of outcomes may exaggerate positive effects and underreport deterioration. Without acknowledging its mixed effects, the field cannot approach the deep ethical problem of costing out its benefits against the price of its liabilities.

Unfortunately, even the more analytic of the reviewers ignore the broader implications of the field's weak scholarship. The problem of testing the outcomes of social welfare programs, especially those delivered in the "clinical" style, is not simply one of appropriate method, but also includes the commitment to deploy that method fairly—that is, a commitment to tough scrutiny and skepticism. The contentment in the field with weak research and the true-believer style of both its practitioners and researchers hints that family therapy is more a cult of cure than a serious and rational enterprise dedicated to resolving family problems. In comparison with individual therapy, family therapy seems even more millenarian, marginal, and unresponsive to scientific standards of proof.

The failure of family therapy may arise in the first instance from its faulty basic assumptions. The family may not be an appropriate focus for the treatment of family problems. Family therapy seems to overstate the independence of the family from its social setting, as though families, especially dysfunctional ones, were capable of walling off the influence of the broader culture and providing a refuge for its members from the stresses of life. To the contrary, families may be dysfunctional precisely because the tensions they cause their members express problems in the secular organizations of society. Family members may bring home their problems. The structure of intrafamily functioning, the core locus for family intervention, may not be as mutually interdependent as it is dependent upon forces outside of the family. Without acknowledging the influence of those broader institutions, it may be impossible to address problems within the family.

The social history of modern life is the story of the declining influence of the nuclear and extended families in deference to the marketplace, the workplace, the school, television and other organs of mass communication, and the peer group. The modern notion of the civic culture that underpins contemporary democratic society is an acknowledgment of this shift. Relative to the ideal family of American autarchy and even in contrast to the preindustrial family, the modern nuclear family provides a relatively small amount of socialization for its members. Therefore, the reliance of family therapy upon obsolete notions of family independence may produce the impossibly romantic task of treating a follower as if it were a leader, a symptom as if it were a cause, and an expression as if it were the inspiration itself.

This romantic belief in the possibility of family preservation through psychotherapy has had cruel effects. As long as family therapy is seen as effective, family interventions are justified for dysfunctional families with the effect that reasonable alternatives, including family dissolution, are delayed or ignored. As one example, protective foster placements for abused and neglected children are deferred as family therapy is applied to preserve dysfunctional families. However, in some cases at least, the reluctance to dissolve dysfunctional families in favor of foster care has had tragic effects that could have probably been prevented with a more realistic assessment of the efficacy of family psychotherapy.[3]

Secondly, the family system may not be amenable to manipulation. Family psychotherapy, especially in its typically weak form of some ten or fifteen hours of discussion with a therapist, may have greatly exaggerated the degree to which human behavior is amenable to change, especially reasoned change. The behaviors of dysfunctional families may be deeply embedded habits—not just the stylistic failures of individual family members—that are actually reinforced through their roles in broader cultural institutions. An oppressive male dominance within a family may express the values of a subculture and may not be amenable to change without changing the subculture itself. The personality disorders of parents may have been permanently imprinted in their own families of birth and reinforced in a variety of work situations that reward unchained aggression and compulsiveness, as two examples, with status and salary. The modern family may not provide an adequate avenue through which to correct these behaviors since it probably does not control a sufficient area of an individual's psychological environment. Indeed, divorce itself may emerge when the family becomes incompatible with broader cultural institutions, such as work, and broader cultural values, such as financial success.

But whatever the potential merits of speculations about the nature of family dysfunction, the family therapy literature has not even begun to amass any credible evidence to support its underlying theories. Indeed, its failures of proof suggest that the tenets of family therapy may be fundamentally marred. The practice of family therapy has failed to dispel the skeptic's observation that by the time the dysfunctions of a family are recognized, it seems likely that they will not be corrected by the weak, inexpensive, and superficial interventions of a family therapist.

Curiously, family therapy may be most useful when the family is *not* the principal mediator of a member's problem, as for example, in the case of biologically determined individual conditions such as schizophrenia and autism. In these cases, family therapy teaches family members to adjust most effectively to the behaviors of its dysfunctional member in a manner that minimizes symptoms. But in these cases, family therapy is not therapy at all; it acts largely as a neutral information source in the same way as a visiting nurse teaches one spouse to care for the stroke of the other spouse.

In the end, family psychotherapy, just like individual psychotherapy, does not appear to have a demonstrable production function. Its theoretical underpinnings are weakened enormously by their inability to inspire effective intervention. Most discouraging, the field lacks a scholarly community that is dedicated to the search for demonstrable remedies. Yet despite its apparent uselessness as a corrective for personal and social problems, family therapy may endure to reinforce dominant social values, although paradoxically not the family values that justify is apparent utility. In this curious way, the field achieves its social sanction by denying its ostensible commitment to assist families in trouble.

Similar to individual psychotherapy, family psychotherapy endorses the possibility of a socially efficient domestic policy, the idea that inexpensive and culturally compatible interventions are adequate correctives for serious social problems. Family therapy provides the comforting notion that socialization can be inexpensively purchased through restored families. Families after all are fundamentally voluntary relationships in which the largest amount of caring is provided by unpaid caregivers. Expensive alternatives to voluntary care, especially in light of large federal deficits and other competing social priorities, are politically repugnant.

In denying the abiding force of social institutions outside of the family, a psychotherapeutic focus on the individual within the family buttresses the culture's preference to isolate individual responsibility from its social context. In contrast, a greater recognition of social causation—the notion that individual behavior is a product of experiences that the broader society has a responsibility to provide—would tend to justify the public provision of surrogate institutions for failed families (e.g., foster care, schooling, jobs, and so forth).

Notes

1. The following randomized studies of family therapy were not analyzed simply because their inadequacies are redundant with the studies that are cited and discussed: Baucom, Sayers, and Sher 1990; Bowers and Al-Redha 1990; Clarkin et al. 1990; Friedman 1989; Glick et al. 1985; Haas et al. 1988; Huber and Milstein 1985; Lieberman, Weston, and Pawl 1991; Raue and Spence 1985; Saarijarvi, Rytokoski and Alanen 1991; Saarijarvi et al. 1992; Waring et al. 1990; Waring et al. 1991; Zweben, Pearlman, and Li 1988. In all, during the thirteen years from 1980 through 1992 there appear to be fewer than fifty randomized studies in all of psychotherapy.
2. Azrin et al. 1980; Boelens et al. 1980; Cobb et al. 1984; Girodo, Stein, and Dotzenroth 1980; O'Leary 1981; Hahlweg et al. 1982; Mehlman, Baucom, and Anderson 1983; Szapocznik et al. 1983; Brock and Joanning 1983; Jacobson 1984; O'Farrell, Cutter, and Floyd 1985; Johnson and Greenberg 1985; Baucom and Lester 1986; Holtzworth-Monroe, Jacobson, and Deklyen 1989; Jacobson et al. 1989; Snyder and Wills 1989; Behrens, Sanders, and Halford 1990; Baucom, Sayers, and Sher 1990; Snyder, Wills, and Grady-Fletcher 1991.
3. The failure of a strategy of family preservation for a foster care population has been measured in one of the rare strong studies of any intervention. It provides a very suggestive view of family therapy itself. See Schuerman et al. 1993; Schuerman et al. 1994.

5

The Failure of Psychotherapy as Science

This review of the best outcome research in psychotherapy—individual, group, and family—leads to a conclusion about the "ordinary" methods of psychotherapy that are virtually identical with the National Academy of Sciences' conclusions relative to biofeedback, training, extrasensory perception, and the other "extraordinary," "unconventional" methods of enhancing human performance. There is not one credible, definitive test of the value of individual and group therapy or marital therapy. There is no credible replication of any research. The methodological and scholarly inadequacies of psychotherapy outcome research set the entire psychotherapeutic enterprise outside of science. The literature's susceptibility to subjectivity and a host of biases suggests that the field has constructed a defensive narrative for professional advantage rather than an objective, scientific estimate of psychotherapy's effectiveness. The scientific level of inquiry in psychotherapy is still immature, producing a professionally self-serving body of emotion covered in the robes of science. Paradoxically the field's vulgarized research exemplifies the postmodern critique—subservience to social power—even while it is itself a victim of the weaknesses of postmodern forms of research.

The very human tendency of practitioners to press for evidence of their effectiveness has been given free reign in the field, overwhelming the modest and inadequate methodological protections of the research. In spite of the recent appetite for randomized designs, the body of outcome research falls into an embarrassment of methodological pitfalls, ultimately failing to exclude a host of alternative explanations for the reported results. It is even likely that the reported outcomes are obscuring consistent patient deterioration, once again reprising the most troublesome of all criticisms of the therapeutic enterprise. Still and all, the frail commitment of the field to minimal standards of scientific publication has allowed for the reinterpretation of its reported findings. This is no small achievement.

Methods and Interventions

With few exceptions, the body of psychotherapy research tested minimal interventions on small groups of patients. Reflecting the society's impatience with drawn-out and expensive treatments, the interventions were typically short-term, usually a few months and frequently just a few treatments; consisted of short sessions, usually one to two hours per week; and involved few caregivers and a small amount of physical resources.

More importantly, the interventions rarely carried a reasonable theoretical presumption of effectiveness into the research situation. On the surface, it seemed quite implausible that a few hours of exhortation, the core of most therapies, would be capable of changing embedded behaviors. But the prior research itself, customarily cited as a justification for the experiment, had typically failed to establish the merit of the intervention and never through adequate research methodologies. More often than not a social imperative (e.g., the seriousness of juvenile delinquency or the cost of care) and not any prior clinical evidence justified the experiment.

The studies almost uniformly failed to protect against the expectancy biases of researchers and clinicians; patients may often have been subtly induced to mimic improved behaviors without having actually changed their own problem behaviors. Many patients may have felt a loyalty to the research project and a special gratitude or affection for their therapists. Their reports of personal behavior change, especially at follow-up, may have suppressed failures that they felt would damage the project or affect their standing in their therapists' eyes. For the same reasons, they may have exaggerated their improvements.

Blinding, an important protection against biased assessment, was infrequent while outcome data were usually drawn from patients by raters—researchers, therapists, and their students—whose careers were caught up with the success of the research project. Even where the research claimed that evaluators were blind, cues to the subject's status were probably provided by the subjects themselves in interviews or the cues may have been evident in the video- and audiotapes that were often employed to rate patient behaviors; verbal or physical patient responses may have signaled whether the patient was in an experimental or control group as well as the type of therapy that was administered.

In addition to the likelihood of biased raters, serious inadequacies flawed many of the measurement instruments in almost every study. Few raters were employed, preventing adequate tests of reliability. Measures infrequently reached highly reliable levels while some studies utilized clearly unreliable measures. The validity of measurement was also a common problem.

While subjects were frequently randomized between control groups and experimental groups, the controls themselves were usually inadequate to establish the importance of the therapeutic intervention. Typically, the research employed standard treatment controls, and in the absence of evidence that the standard treatment was effective, the status of the experimental outcomes was difficult to estimate.

In addition, the common reliance upon wait-list controls may not be useful since patients may seek care while on the wait list; they may deteriorate because they are on the wait list; they may simply disappear from the study; or, the greatest challenge to the value of the research, the fact of being wait-listed may distort their reporting behavior.

Placebo controls and nontreatment controls were rarely utilized. As a result, the efficacy of therapy itself could not be tested.

Besides randomized control groups and unbiased measurement, many other necessary precautions to assure credibility were not employed. Control and experimental groups usually numbered less than thirty subjects; samples of less than twenty were common. Small samples are more susceptible than large samples to bias; they also threaten representativeness and the comparability between groups. Moreover, the size of outcome differences required to reach statistical significance increases as the size of the sample shrinks; this imposes greater demands on the power of the intervention, while perhaps tempting greater rater bias.

Subjects were never randomly selected from the underlying population that suffered from the psychological debility. Based upon self-selected patients and convenience samples, the results of the studies may not represent the broader social problem of psychological distress that justified the research in the first place.

The experiments were typically conducted under demonstration conditions that may have taken advantage of extraordinary motivations among staff and researchers to produce positive effects. Failing to replicate the common conditions under which therapy is delivered, the studies became statements of optimal care. Indeed, any therapeutic gains in these kinds of situations cannot be attributed to therapy itself but to the possibly unique concern of the therapists or the unique degree of scrutiny under which they worked. In this case, extraordinary human caring or close surveillance, not the routinized processes of psychotherapy, may have accounted for the gains, a very unhappy conclusion for the professional aspirations of the field.

Follow-up measures were rarely taken at appropriate lengths of time after therapy. Typically, follow-up evaluations, if they were made, took place within a few months after therapy. In the absence of credible follow-up data, the extended effects of therapy cannot be established.

The statistical procedures of the research were sometimes inappropriate, even though this was often the strongest suit of many studies. With small samples, the differences between control and experimental groups need to be very large in order to achieve statistical significance. Nevertheless, large initial differences that are not yet statistically significant between experimental groups and controls may illegitimately contribute to statistically significant outcome differences. Researchers rarely estimated the degree to which these initial differences accounted for their outcomes. Moreover, adjustments in significance levels for repeated comparisons were rarely made.

In short, the methodological imperfections of the studies vitiated any ability to answer their defining research questions. The pointlessness of most studies raises an ethical concern in pestering patients to participate in research of little theoretical or practical importance.

Outcomes

The most frequently reported research outcomes were positive and modest. Yet, taken together the findings are interpreted by the individual authors and the field generally as evidence that psychotherapy is broadly and consistently effective against a great number of serious psychological and social problems. In addition, the research commends the growing efficiency of the field for developing shorter-term and, therefore, less costly treatments that are as effective as their lengthier predecessors. With rare exceptions, the authors accepted the credibility of their findings in spite of the deficiencies of their methods. The authors of many meta-analyses even went so far as to applaud the progress of the psychotherapeutic enterprise both in terms of its growing clinical power as well as its scholarly sophistication.

Yet, the field's conclusions exaggerated both the clinical and theoretical importance of the research. Its many serious methodological deficiencies opened the door to alternative explanations of the findings. Expectancy biases, measurement imperfections, patient misreports, researcher errors, demonstration effects, and selection biases may more accurately account for the reported positive advantages of psychotherapy than any beneficial power of the therapy itself.

In the end, the relative effectiveness of psychotherapy in comparison with either natural remission or sustained structural solutions for social problems—an alternative that is plausible on its face and that enjoys a long scholarly tradition of support—has not been demonstrated. The small and frequently trivial advantages of psychotherapy over its own imperfect controls are lost against the background of the scholarship's methodological static.

Psychotherapy has still not demonstrated its effectiveness. The extended impact of this failure is to deny the plausibility of a strategy of social efficiency within the context of contemporary American social problems. Indeed, the consistent indeterminacy of psychotherapy's benefits beg for reconsideration of alternatives to socially efficient solutions—the broad-based provision of adequate social institutions.

Yet, the most troubling implication of the research is not simply that psychotherapy is an inadequate substitute for deeper institutional strategies, but that psychotherapy has no advantage over frank neglect, even reprising the possibility that psychotherapy may actually accelerate the psychological deterioration of many patients without conferring commensurate improvements on others.

Patient Deterioration

Psychotherapy's brief period of skepticism, for perhaps ten years starting in the mid-1960s, contained a few primary studies that questioned the effectiveness of its outcomes. This handful of studies (Gottshalk et al. 1973; Frank 1973; Park and Covi 1965; Brill 1966; Errera et al. 1967; Strupp 1972; and perhaps a few others) and a reprisal of Eysenck's earlier work raised a series of methodological and substantive questions about the credibility of psychotherapy's outcomes and the effectiveness of the field's techniques. They pointed out that untreated patients frequently did as well as treated patients, that symptoms tended to subside naturally ("spontaneous remission"), that patients receiving placebo treatments frequently did as well as and sometimes better than those receiving therapy, and that relatively healthy patients—the worried well—were frequently the subjects of psychotherapy that was initially intended for far sicker people.[1] Most troubling of all, however, was the suggestion that many patients may actually have deteriorated as a result of therapy, that therapy itself may be harmful.

A number of more recent sources of data reaffirm this earlier skepticism. Lambert, Weber, and Sykes (1993) estimated that the placebo effect accounts for much of the reported positive outcomes. Their effect size of .43 (17 percent improvement of a maximum possible improvement of 50 percent or, said another way, patients who receive placebos are better off than 67 percent of controls) sets a minimal hurdle that positive findings must cross before they can be attributed to the therapeutic intervention itself. Rosenthal and Rubin (1978) raised this hurdle even higher by estimating that a huge amount of the reported findings—perhaps as much as a full standard deviation, that is, an effect size of 1.0 (34 percent improvement out of a possible 50 percent)—may be due to expectancy biases. Moreover, the possibility of expectancy bias increases as the research becomes methodologically more porous.

However, the Smith, Glass, and Miller (1980) enterprise, based upon very compromised research, reported therapeutic benefits of only .85 (30.2 percent improvement; those treated are better off than 80.2 percent of controls), far less than the combination of placebo effects and expectancy biases. Even acknowledging some overlap between the estimates of placebo effects and expectancy biases, the tyranny of group data (the direct implication of parametric assumptions) suggests that many, if not most patients do not improve in therapy. Indeed, many patients probably deteriorate. Moreover, the size of the deterioration may be very large, approaching 50 percent for many therapies in light of the reinterpreted data of Smith, Glass, and Miller (1980). Outcomes that are this dispersed imply a Wild West of psychotherapeutic outcomes and not the carefully engineered cures that the literature suggests. Yet, very few studies after Smith, Glass, and Miller (1980) reported any positive findings that exceeded the hurdle of expectancy bias and placebo effects. Most positive findings, produced by methodologically suspect studies, fell far short, while the few instances of reported deterioration raise profoundly disturbing questions.

The field's estimates of its effectiveness have been inflated by many more factors—measurement bias, selection bias, and so forth—than expectancy biases alone. The possibility of actual degeneration in therapy reprises itself forcefully; if outcome data could somehow be adjusted for these biases, then an immense amount of deterioration in therapy might be displayed. Deterioration in therapy may not be all that surprising since people with emotional problems, especially in confronting those problems, may get worse. Moreover, since much of mental illness is adaptive to a dysfunctional social milieu, the psychotherapeutic process of confronting emotional problems, together with its inability to directly affect conditions outside of the treatment room, may frustrate and exacerbate already disturbed patients.

Therapy may not be a benign process and its harms may be very costly. The therapeutic process is open to all sorts of abuses. Therapist abuses (Masson 1988), such as predations on the vulnerabilities of patients and maintaining ineffective but remunerative therapies, may be abundant but institutional abuses may be both more common and more serious. At its core, patient deterioration may also result from the therapist's deep attachment to techniques of cure, prevention, and rehabilitation that are simply not effective. As a result of an institutional refusal to conduct fair tests of its outcomes, psychotherapeutic practice may have developed an institutional blindness to the possibility of its own harmful techniques. Ineffectiveness may be the toxic by-product of the field's distortion of its scientific commitments.

Still, without adequate epidemiological estimates of the natural course of mental illness and without appropriate controls, the deterioration of patients in therapy cannot be tied to the psychotherapeutic interventions themselves. Yet the burden for proving effectiveness and safety rests with the therapeutic community, and, especially in light of a presumable basis of deterioration, not with the skeptic.

Psychotherapy's compromise of its research has been the result of its worldly obedience to contemporary American society. The acquiescence of its intellectual life and its isolation from the needs of less privileged social groups suggest that its role in clinical care may not be its central function. Rather, psychotherapy creates some of the myths that the nation lives by, reinforcing the comforting belief that minimal expenditures on one form of moral suasion or another are adequate to repair the damage caused by deep institutional deprivations.

Psychotherapy is not a young discipline anymore. It has been intensively pursued as a clinical practice for over sixty years—far longer than many specialties in the natural sciences and in medicine. Its longstanding failure to apply rigorous methodologies to its outcomes cannot be attributed to the absence of appropriate methodologies; randomized placebo controls are feasible, ethical, and legal. Rather, the absence of credible tests of the effectiveness of psychotherapy results from a stubborn avoidance of independent scrutiny. Psychotherapy has been able to withstand clinical accountability on the strength of its social and political activities, particularly its endorsement of regnant cultural values through myths of socially efficient cures for societal problems.

If scientific credibility was the goal of research funding, then the government, particularly through the National Institute of Mental Health (and many private donors, frequently philanthropic foundations), have wasted a lot of money. However, if they wanted objectivity then their canny administrators certainly would not have given the evaluation dollars to the very people being evaluated. It seems far more reasonable that funding for research is knowingly a subsidy for convenient myth.

The Subcommunity of Psychotherapy Researchers

The wide acceptance of critical research in the hard sciences and in engineering explains a large portion of their success. But precisely because the culture does not insist upon the same sort of rigor for psychotherapy as it does for drugs, surgery and medicine, buildings, bridges, roads, cars, dishwashers, and airplanes, the porous methods of postmodernism have established estates within the psychotherapy subcommunity. Obviously, the culture is not as concerned about the production functions of psychotherapy—cure, prevention, and rehabilitation—as it is with its social functions.

Psychotherapy and social services generally have undermined scientific rigor with an enthusiasm for "practical" postmodern methodologies: single subject designs (Kratochwill 1978), the case formulation approach (Persons 1991), ethnographic content analysis (Smith, Sells, and Newfield, unpublished), the heuristic paradigm (Heineman Pieper

1989), hermeneutics, and many others. There would be little problem if these techniques were merely employed as preliminary tools of investigation; any source of inspiration is acceptable as long as the inspiration eventually builds to a critical test of its value. However, these weak research designs are consistently graduated to a more definitive status by researchers who claim that they are "widely considered acceptable methods of scientific inquiry" (Silverman 1991, 1351). Nevertheless, conventional use and agreement are not proofs of anything except cultural compatibility.

These postmodern techniques are reversions to more immature scientific forms. They tolerate, even celebrate, many breeches of scientific rigor, lacking controls and safeguards against expectancy biases, accepting practitioner judgments of outcomes, and employing unreliable criteria of outcomes. These regressions in scientific development mark the accommodation of the field with political realities.

The poor scientific quality of the research maintains the myth of social efficiency. The multitude of interlocking institutional relations between the research and the culture are constructed through a series of rewards and punishments—funding, consultantships, appointments, promotions, media exposure, and celebrity, but also censorship, isolation, and more material penalties—that induce supposedly neutral research projects to endorse social preferences.

Psychotherapy has broken its commitments to objective research in deference to a far more profitable role in sustaining contemporary myth—social efficiency. It has become another bauble on a timeless string of superstition and spectral truths that undermine rational impulses in public life and the promise of a humane civic culture.

The Lost Commitment

The consistent failure of psychotherapy research to perform critical tests of its effectiveness signals a lost resolve in the portion of the scientific community that investigates psychotherapy. It is also broadly suggestive, especially in light of the resources placed into this research over time, of a distortion in the operations of the culture that subverts the defining tasks of that subcommunity.

The small critical tradition has not prevailed in either the subcommunity of psychotherapy researchers nor more broadly in the social services. Very few have had the courage to broadly question the effectiveness of psychotherapy and its social meaning: Eysenck (1965), Rachman (1971), the early Bergin (1971), Gross (1978), Rieff (1966), perhaps Truax and Carkhuff (1967), Prioleau, Murdock, and Brody (1983), and a few others. In the social services, the critical tradition has been even more constricted: Wootton (1959), the early Fischer (1973), the young Cloward (Cloward and Epstein 1967), Martinson (1974), Sechrest, White, and Brown, eds. (1979), Epstein (1993) and very few more.

Especially in light of the postmodern belief that the "monument" of culture induces intellectual obedience and social conformity, it is worth emphasizing that the small amount of deep questioning took place in psychotherapy during a general period of institutional challenge, the 1960s and early 1970s. The skeptical research itself, imperfect even while occasionally superior to the research it was indicting, may have mediated the spirit of its times through the expectancies and biases of its own researchers. In other periods too, the broader preferences of the society, especially reflected in its intellectual life, seem to have been played out through the psychotherapy literature. During a period of doubt, the field expressed the culture's skepticism toward the effectiveness of established institutions, but during a period of credulity and belief, the more customary condition of society, the field conformed with the dictates of stability.

Yet it is easy to exaggerate the weight of skepticism during even the brief period of doubt. During this time, perhaps ten challenges to the reigning orthodoxy of the field's effectiveness appeared in a literature that probably contained well over 20,000 journal articles. Moreover, these few challenges did not decisively settle any issue, being in their own right open to a number of methodological challenges.

Since the brief period of doubt that seemed to have been dispelled by the Smith et al. enterprise (Glass 1976; Smith and Glass 1977; Smith, Glass, and Miller 1980), criticism, when it occurred at all, usually emerged in the conflicts among therapeutic factions and rarely spilled over into a form that questioned the very nature of the therapeutic enterprise itself. When methodological problems were discussed (Rosenthal's many comments as examples), they were hardly ever applied in a systematic review to the quality of the field's information. Rather, these types of immensely sophisticated and frequently arcane discussions were muted, isolated, partialized, and, in the end, ineffectual in pressing the necessary issues of effectiveness itself. When a weak study appeared that supported the field's ambitions, its faults were sometimes noted but its findings quickly entered the mantra of the field's happy meditations.

Customarily too, the issue of the field's social meaning was divorced from the issue of its effectiveness. Critics tended to find fault because therapists were not seeing many in need or because the field reinforced an unjust status quo. These were safe faults, testimony that psychotherapy should be made more universally available and that the field should gain greater professional independence. Still, there have been few penetrating analyses of psychotherapy's social role through the lens of its clinical effectiveness.

The absence of appropriate criticism is a problem of the scholarly subcommunity in psychotherapy itself, its inhospitality to criticism, its insistence on effectiveness. Yet the psychotherapeutic community has no apparent motive to pursue the question of its effectiveness. The broader intellectual culture has not produced a corrective challenge—neither funds for independent replications nor much scholarly discussion of the possibility of psychotherapy's failures. The truth-seeking function of science has been subordinated to the social role of psychotherapy. Professional ambitions have connived with dominant social interests to propagate the fiction of psychotherapy's clinical effectiveness in support of the myth of social efficiency.

The age picks its philosophy. Science has not been the culprit in the unfortunate consequences of a widespread belief in social efficiency. Psychotherapy's folk tales of rational induction and virtuous control have prevailed because they appeal to a sufficiently large constituency. But having found a convenience in the postmodern apology for self-absorption and social indifference, these social actors are undermining the civic virtues of a more scientific culture through the myths of psychotherapeutics.

Note

1. Garfield provides a standard response to Eysenck's recent discussion of patient deterioration and the ineffectiveness of psychotherapy (both in Dryden and Feltham 1992). Garfield's argument rests upon the power of placebo conditions. He holds that they have powerful effects, but he insists that these effects are psychotherapeutic containing "a number of the factors that are common to most of the psychotherapies" (128). This is similar to Kleinman's position that "psychotherapy may very well be a way of maximizing placebo responses, a nonspecific treatment effect, but if so, it should be applauded, rather than condemned, for exploiting a useful therapeutic process which is underutilized in general health

care" (Kleinman 1988, 112). However, the problem for psychotherapy is to demonstrate the value that it adds to patient optimism (the expectation of cure) that results from common time structured activities provided by nontherapists and furthermore to demonstrate that long-term clinical value of these nonspecific factors. Proof that psychotherapy adds little to common human kindness or to simple social activities—that it does not build on placebo responses and that it may in essence be little more than a placebo response—invalidates the professional utility of the field. Garfield further relies upon the four decades of research since Eysenck's 1952 research to come to the conclusion that psychotherapy is generally effective. Previous chapters have addressed this issue. Frank and Frank (1991) also fail to provide a convincing endorsement for placebo effects as true therapeutic outcomes—credibly measured, meaningful in resolving the presenting distress, and sustained over time—while their reading of the literature itself is both selective and tendentious, citing research that supports their arguments, but avoiding the scientific limitations of the evidence itself. Furthermore, the parallel they draw between faith healing—the priest function and Torrey's witch doctor—and the placebo effect in psychotherapy does not validate therapy itself without credible proof of the latter's efficacy and the ability of psychotherapy to produce it with regularity. The priest function as the essential therapeutic role also raises serious ethical issues of paternalistically mislabeling faith as science; but this is a separate topic.

6

Conclusion: Why Does Psychotherapy Persist?

"The question... is not whether psychotherapy works; that goes without saying."
—Frank and Frank 1991, xiv

The voice of science in the psychotherapy community is weak, lacking any apparent influence over the quality of its research or the depth of its self-scrutiny. The scholarship of psychotherapy more resembles the intensely censored communication of cults than the open, direct, and tough cross-examining challenges that define intellectual exchanges between scholars committed to the canons of science. The field's poor research masks patient deterioration and protects its communal interests at the expense of the broader civic culture. Critical thought itself seems to have largely abandoned the therapeutic enterprise. The compatibility between an ineffective practice of psychotherapy and the larger stakes in social efficiency suggests that the society is content with the ineffable benefits of psychotherapy, its generation of myth.

The contemporary orthodoxy of psychotherapeutic effectiveness, most recently restated by Bergin and Garfield (1994), is largely unchallenged:

> There is little doubt that psychological treatments are, overall and in general, beneficial, although it remains equally true that not everyone benefits to a satisfactory degree. (144)
>
> Psychologists, psychiatrists, social workers, and marriage and family therapists, as well as patients can be assured that a broad range of therapies, when offered by skillful, wise and stable therapists, are likely to result in appreciable gains for the client. (180)

Hardly any critic of psychotherapy is willing to conclude that its social role is devoid of a rational clinical function. Even Eysenck backed away from this conclusion, stressing that the benefits of psychotherapy may be offset by patient deterioration. Fortunately for his commitment to psychiatry, Eysenck discovered virtue in behavioral therapy. Kline (in Dryden and Feltham 1992) only acknowledged that psychotherapy's outcomes were indeterminate. Dawes, while criticizing the field's scientific basis in a manner similar to Kline and concluding that the benefits of psychotherapy are greatly exaggerated, still found occasional value in a number of psychotherapeutic interventions (Dawes 1994, 73). In his turn, Kline (1988) reserves a value for psychotherapy to prod people to take action against their problems, even while accepting science as an appropriate method for its evaluation (147).

Nevertheless, the deficient scholarship of the field constitutes a fable of what happens when a commitment to science is betrayed. The effectiveness of psychotherapy, grossly exaggerated by its literature, is at best indeterminate, the conclusion that flows ineluctably from the scientific scrutiny of its outcome studies. However, it is a more reasonable surmise that psychotherapy is ineffective and perhaps even routinely harmful. If the body of research is to be taken on its own terms, then patient deterioration must be accepted as a consistent finding of primary studies. Moreover, the many meta-analyses, particularly Smith, Glass, and Miller (1980), display a normal distribution of effect sizes across those primary studies that implies many negative outcomes (and an enormous amount of deterioration to the extent to which the Smith, Glass, and Miller standard deviations are standard errors). These estimates of negative effects are certainly too low since the positive findings, small to begin with after adjustment for placebo effects, are inflated by a variety of biases, particularly expectancy bias, and a host of other self-serving imperfections in the study procedures. Additional adjustments for these imperfections would move the normal curve of outcomes further into the area of negative results.

Yet deterioration would seem to be conjectural since there has not actually been credible proof of the ineffectiveness of psychotherapy. While patient deterioration is documented by a few studies, these studies are no more rigorous than those that document positive outcomes. Nevertheless, the conjectures of harm are at least as sound as the best research in the field. These conjectures define an important point of skepticism that a large portion and perhaps even the net effect of psychotherapy may be harmful. Yet the scholarly literature of the field and the society itself have simply ignored the persistent possibility of ineffectiveness and harm, thus quietly shifting the traditional burden of proof from the shoulders of the clinician to the shoulders of the skeptic. The profession of psychotherapy—its practice and theory—are apparently disciplined by considerations other than its clinical effectiveness.

Harm in psychotherapy may result from three sources. First, the utilization of psychotherapy may delay or subvert the provision of effective remedies. Patients may deteriorate during the course of ineffective psychotherapy. Many mental and emotional problems may subside only by changing the patient's environment. These alternatives—safe havens and surrogate care—are customarily more expensive than psychotherapy. In these cases, the belief in the efficacy of psychotherapy thwarts the provision of alternative remedies. Szasz's comment about psychoanalysis is relevant to psychotherapy and social therapeutics generally:

> The poor need jobs and money, not psychoanalysis. The uneducated need knowledge and skills, not psychoanalysis. Furthermore, the poor and the uneducated are also often politically disfranchised and socially oppressed; if this is the case, they need freedom from oppression. The kind of *personal* freedom that psychoanalysis promises can have meaning only for persons who enjoy a large measure of economic, political, and social freedom. (Szasz 1965, 28)

Secondly, psychotherapy itself, even under optimal conditions—when it is provided by trained therapists who employ appropriate techniques—may be harmful. The process of self-scrutiny may simply be inappropriate and counterproductive for the emotional problems of even well-heeled people. Psychotherapy's brave assumptions about man's rational capacities may produce treatments that abrade many troubled people, denying them the solace of self-deceit, and fostering a series of disruptive social behaviors.

Third, optimal conditions may be consistently scorned by unscrupulous, incompetent, or immoral practitioners. Therapist improprieties may be prevalent. The structure for delivering psychotherapeutic care (private practice and professional autonomy), for training practitioners, and for regulating services may not be capable of remedying these deficiencies. The market interests of practitioners may produce a feckless form of psychotherapy that insidiously continues both the patients' self-love and their course of therapy rather than addressing their true needs. Some patients become addicted to psychotherapy, recalling Pallone's (1986) wry construction of a self-perpetuating psychotherapeutic marketplace in which the goals of one school of therapy are the treatable symptoms for another.

Psychotherapy, far from releasing the soul of man from the confines of an unjust and suffocating tradition, has failed to professionalize either compassion or an effective remedy for deviant behavior. Its research has offered no credible evidence that distinguishes psychotherapy as more effective than the popular psychotherapies, the multitude of self-help regimens, and placebo treatments. Rather, the field has created fictions of effectiveness that deprive those in need of a just advocacy. Psychotherapy's socially efficient cures have become the conditions of citizenship for many lower status and poor Americans. By producing the myths that reconcile the disadvantaged to their fates, the field has become one of the principal apologists for contemporary society.

Psychotherapy's failure as science, a sacrifice of knowledge to power, has nurtured a cultic milieu of subjectivity and implicit truth in which political compatibility conveniently supplants rigorous controlled experimentation as the test of service effectiveness. In protection of its privileged social position, the field has courted a barren marriage of the therapist's self-interest and the society's resistance to redistributional impulses. Weaker derivative fields—social work, counseling, educational psychology, and criminology—have adapted the myths of psychotherapeutics to their own social problem franchises. The likelihood of the ineffectiveness of psychotherapy and therapeutics generally goes far to suggest that the culture has actually devalued the production function of the social services in deference to their ceremonial function: to promote a generalized theory of social therapeutics that endorses socially efficient but ineffective responses to serious social distress.

In the short run, patient deterioration may be the price of this insistence upon socially efficient remedies. In the longer term, the practice of psychotherapy propagates the inequities of society by providing a mechanism that muffles the voice of deprived groups. In addition to legitimating the harm caused by bogus cures, the contemporary practice of psychotherapy is legitimating hardship.

Alternatives to socially efficient but ineffective remedies are not tenable as long as the belief is firm that therapeutics are effective. A strategy of greater social equality that replicates customary and essential social institutions for those without families, education, jobs, livable communities, and so forth is immensely expensive and, therefore, politically unacceptable. The difficulty of facing the source of America's social problems—money, not personal character—casts a shadow into the next millennium.

The Communal Problem of Psychotherapy

Even the best of the psychotherapy researchers—those with apparent commitments to science—and many of its severest critics seem to be in the thrall of its mythic effectiveness. Rosenthal and Rubin (1978) defined a profound challenge to the effectiveness of psychotherapy by demonstrating the plausibility of expectancy effects in psychology research, notably psychophysiological research. Nevertheless, their comments concluded with loyal testimony to the effectiveness of psychotherapy:

> Thus there is now abundant evidence that aspirin and psychotherapy are causally-effective treatments for particular dependent variables, even though the precise mechanisms responsible for these causal effects are not known. (1978)

Rosenthal and Rubin (1978) accepted the early evidence of the Smith, Glass, and Miller (1980) meta-analysis (initially reported in Smith and Glass 1977). Paradoxically, at the same time that Rosenthal and Rubin (1978) were conceding their skepticism to the evidence produced by this meta-analysis (Smith and Glass 1977), Smith, Glass, and Miller (1980) themselves provided additional data that seemed to support Rosenthal and Rubin's (1978) initial doubts. In their 1980 book, Smith, Glass, and Miller reported that the reactivity of measures (the degree to which measures are susceptible to researcher biases), a relative of expectancy bias, accounted for a portion of the positive outcomes in the research that they covered.

In another instance of blind faith among the field's best researchers, Weisz et al. (1990) concluded their evaluation of the Willie M Program with the expectation that more therapy, better matched to the needs of the program participants, would be effective. This study, even though it was prevented by legal constraints from randomizing subjects between control and experimental conditions, was a model of skeptical logic applied to the outcomes of a social service program. Yet, after demonstrating the failure of intensive services to resolve the problems of severely disturbed adolescents, the authors refused to consider the possibility that psychotherapy is simply an ineffective intervention and that effective "treatment" for very deprived youths may have required intensive participation in the normal cultural institutions of the society. In contrast, their evaluation concluded that "what may now remain is the task of identifying specific interventions that are (a) demonstrably effective with these high-risk youth and (b) sufficiently well-defined that they can be applied appropriately by multiple mental health workers in multiple settings" (Weisz et al. 1990).

Even the most technically proficient researchers appear to be incapable of sustaining an appropriate scientific skepticism toward the effectiveness of psychotherapy. The larger portion of the field's intellectual community, and by far the weaker portion, is in hasty retreat from self-doubt. Their credulity raises the more troubling issue of the demand for loyalty and faith that the subcommunity of therapists presses upon their members.

The scientific enterprise in psychotherapy is not scientific except in a trivial and occasionally statistical sense. Researchers and therapists seem motivated to preserve their status and market position by guarding their claims to effectiveness. Claims of psychotherapy's value are routinely published and accepted without deep scrutiny or suspicion. The literature of psychotherapy and the community that creates it punish heresy.

The field is subliminally conscious of its intellectual problems; the small critical tradition has at least been heard if not invited to stay for dinner.[1] The field frequently claims that the issue of its clinical effectiveness has been proved beyond doubt, recalling Rosenthal and Rubin (1978), and Weisz et al. (1990). An effectiveness beyond doubt easily leads to the conclusion that the current task of research is merely to fine tune therapy and improve its efficiency, usually by better matching therapist, therapy, and client. This is the basis of the recent enthusiasm for "appropriate treatment" (Andrews et al. 1990) and differential treatment (Reid and Hanrahan 1982). Unfortunately, the evidence for appropriate treatment and for differential treatment is drawn from a weaker base of "practical" research than the studies that testify to the effectiveness of psychotherapy itself (Epstein 1993).

The assurance of overall effectiveness has a perverse influence in perpetuating the field's bad research. Imperfect research designs, particularly the failure to employ nontreatment and placebo controls, are excused on grounds that it is unethical to withhold effective treatment from patients. Moreover, the field seems to argue that its difficulties in curing occasional types of patients (perhaps addicts, anorectics, and schizophrenics) will eventually be remedied through research; after all, the preponderance of evidence points to effectiveness, which in turn argues for greater investment in treatment and research.

Yet, despite the communal assurances of psychotherapists, the field has failed to substantiate an effective clinical role. Without a true ability to address its defining problems of treating mental illness, the persistence of the field begs to be explained in terms of its social and political utility—its ideological role.

The Role of Psychotherapy

Except for rare skeptical voices, serious criticisms of psychotherapy typically assume its clinical efficacy but take the field to task for its social roles. A variety of critics have maintained that the field's social authority is exercised illegitimately as a coercive force or otherwise as an unwholesome expression of the dominant ethos (Szasz 1965, 1978; Rieff 1966; Gross 1978; Kline 1988; Pallone 1986). Kline (1988) helpfully goes further to detail the ideological influence of psychotherapy:

> It assumes that all is well in society and that if women feel depressed [as one example] there is something wrong with them. Listen to them, we can discover that perhaps there is something wrong with society. (Kline 1988, 147)

When critics acknowledge the weak nature of the field's information, they customarily maintain a faith in its curative ability even if cure is attendant upon a priestly or shamanistic role (Hugh and McSlavney 1983; Torrey 1986; Frank and Frank 1991; Kleinman 1988) or a derivative role approximating friendship (Schofield 1964). The curative ability, Torrey (1986) argues, is shared between psychotherapists and witch doctors who perform essentially equivalent roles that entail

> a shared worldview, the personal qualities of the therapist, the expectations of the client, and an emerging sense of mastery in the client.... To reduce psychotherapy to a shorthand, one can say that it consists of a magnificent mensch (therapist with therapeutic personal qualities) utilizing an edifice complex (client's expectations and emotional arousal) and invoking the principle of Rumpelstiltskin (naming process arising from a shared worldview) to bring about a Superman syndrome (sense of mastery in the client). (Torrey 1986, 231)

The frequent subtheme of hermeneutic, idiographic, and anthropological descriptions of psychotherapy justifies contemporary practice on nonscientific grounds, artfully rejecting the obligation for credible proofs of outcome. In these cases, the door to professional acceptance swings open to admit faith healing—"the curative influence of mind on body" (Frank and Frank 1991, 112)—and placebo or "nonspecific" treatments as remedies for both somatic and psychic distress. Yet, adducing "proofs" of the value of Lourdes (Frank and Frank 1991) or of traditional folk remedies in Chinese society (Kleinman 1988), while perhaps hinting at productive remedies, are not adequate substitutes for rigorous clinical trials. These appeals to exotic authority supplant credible proof in the manner that evidence from the couch, patient self-reports, and therapist evaluations undermine clinical trials.

Nevertheless, a priestly or religious role suggests that the authority of psychotherapy also contains cultural elements in addition to a narrow sanction for clinical activities. The religious role is not simply enacted through the placebos of faith that may have some clinical importance as "a key ritual of our twentieth-century psychological religion":

> It is now obvious that most tenets of...psychotherapy, are Western man's disguise for a new spirituality. It is the educated person's opportunity to practice religion under the cloak of science. It enables us to call on occult powers of healing while appeasing our Western need for a rational underpinning. It makes little difference that each of the psychotherapies has different faith. *It is the faith itself, not the doctrine, that is the healing agent.* (Emphasis in original. Gross 1978, 35)

Thus, social authority is transformed into clinical cure through the faith of patients, explaining the putative efficacy of psychotherapy's clinical role in terms of placebo effects. The authority vested in the psychotherapist by the culture induces a belief in the patient that cure is possible. The possibility of cure itself has salutary effects.

However, neither the effectiveness of this sequence of cure nor any of the more formal candidates for clinical effectiveness has been credibly verified. Neither the shaman nor the psychotherapist can point to credible evidence of cure, prevention, or rehabilitation. In highly consensual and integrated tribal contexts, the shaman's role may appear to the sentimental outsider as a nostalgic ritual of harmony and reaffirmation. Yet, even in the third world this may not be true. Without an ability to cure psychic distress, the reemerging popularity of analytic psychotherapy that Kleinman (1988) reports in China may signal the increasing disruption of that society—the confrontation of individualism and Confucianism—and not a discovery of more satisfying social forms.

While the field clearly exhibits the normative functions of a religion, and even some of the characteristics of a cult, its role is played out more directly in the political arena as a partisan voice attempting to affect the strategic attitudes underpinning social policy.[2] The organizations of institutionalized psychotherapy proselytize particular values through its clinics, hospitals, research and teaching institutions, journals, professional organizations, and so forth. This role as a moral authority may serve many purposes: to judge the limits of acceptable personal behavior, to sanction deviance by dispensing a variety of inducements and punishments, and to symbolize social reason and social authority.[3]

Psychotherapy loses its anthropological charm, especially in the often violent context of modern society's fierce struggle over limited resources. In the culture of the United States and among industrialized nations generally, the popularity of psychotherapy may carry the implication of coercion in Szasz's and Rieff's narrow sense as well as the denial of social need in a broader sense. Without a true clinical production function, the field's role is shaped more by the ideological requirements of live politics than by the ethical quests of a religion.[4]

Even while the therapeutic process as a clinical intervention may have no more impact than any other religious act, its social meaning may be far more profound. Psychotherapy is not merely a religion, but one of contemporary society's favored social ideologies, one of its principal voices for creating "an aura of sacredness and belief." But in true mythic fashion, the credo of individuality is more hortatory than real; vested in moral suasion and not matched with programmatic investments in education, families, communities, and jobs; focused on wealthy worriers and not taken widely to include impoverished and deprived populations. In this way, psychotherapy may have become a politically valuable conceit of the comfortable, assuaging their philosophic neuroses with the luxury of a purchased friendship (Schofield 1964).

Psychotherapy, Social Services, and Social Efficiency

Psychotherapy is the quintessential program of social efficiency, proffering relatively inexpensive and culturally compatible solutions for deep social problems. The effectiveness of psychotherapeutic techniques provides the core rationale for social work, for counseling, for programs to prevent and reduce crime, juvenile delinquency, and addiction to drugs and alcohol, for social rehabilitation, for recreational "therapy," and, naturally, for the huge number of mental health and hygiene programs that purport to alleviate and to manage mental disease, to reduce psychic anguish, and to enhance personal performance and creativity.

> As a social policy strategy, psychotherapy promises not only to change (cure, prevent and rehabilitate) problem behaviors but to do so cheaply and without disrupting the comfortable flow of society. In a small number of short sessions that do not entail large public expenditures or taxes, that do not imply dislocations of populations, social conflicts, family disruptions, or violence, that do not require major initiatives of planning and implementation, psychotherapy promises to resolve social problems on schedule, in the comfort of an office, and largely by talking. Family therapy and group therapy even offer the benefits of scale. (Epstein 1993, 41)

As organized representations of the relationships between different strata of society, social services have become powerful propagators of socially efficient myths. The impact of these services on social problems are also measures of social progress. Moreover, because they are frequently delivered through a large number of decentralized organizations that are characteristically under the auspices of local boards of community elites, they are the fertile gardens in which myths of social interaction are nourished and dispersed. Social service agencies are important vehicles of community education and social ideology.

Yet, by insisting that cheap progress is possible against prior deprivations, psychotherapeutic research and the social sciences, generally, tend to reduce the gravity of social inequality, insinuating that the material disparities between groups are only weakly associated with grave social consequences and, by implication, that the ineffable qualities of character are the decisive determinants of social outcomes. The logic of this position unfolds in supporting a social policy that promotes character building activities instead of generously underwriting access to basic social institutions for the entire membership of the culture. Tenaciously holding onto moral exhortation at the expense of scientific wisdom, contemporary psychotherapy obediently fulfills this social imperative to implicate personal attributes in place of social conditions as the culprit in individual failure.

Through the creation of myth, the field transcends the confining issue of its clinical effectiveness to compete in broader arenas as a political actor. This participation leads to a sublime contract through which the psychotherapeutic community accepts a franchise for its treatment programs and professional activities and in return provides reassuring evidence that socially efficient approaches are viable. However, to the extent to which a socially efficient strategy continues unjust deprivations, the pact between psychotherapist and society becomes a Faustian bargain.

Because the socially efficient myth of psychotherapy is widely believed, therapy is generally viewed as effective and the appropriate response to need. Failure in therapy is thus attributed to the patient's resistance and not to the inadequacy of social responses to need. What may begin as a neutral diagnosis that impersonal events (a probabilistic environment working through heredity) have conspired to produce unfortunate patient behaviors works itself through a cultural logic—the processes of political competition over scarce resources—to place the locus of failure in the patient's moral, social, civic, and genetic imperfections. This sort of logic relieves the society of an obligation to search further for remedies. As a social convenience, the heat of attention is deflected from the therapist, the scholarly process, and the inadequacies of social arrangements.

As a consequence, the practice of psychotherapy far more than medicine, law, engineering, business, education, or even social work, is to an enormous extent accountable only to itself—to the therapist and to the therapeutic community. Scrutiny of that community through outcome research, or for that matter, scrutiny of any kind, depends upon the permission of therapist and therapeutic program. Without blood oaths of brotherhood, an independent researcher is usually quarantined from practice.

Frank abuses of practice—sexual, professional, and financial—may be underreported. Still, the more important institutional abuses of the therapeutic enterprise—misdirected efforts, abandonment of responsibility, professionally self-serving priorities, and professionally convenient systems of care such as the private clinic and solo practice—probably cause more social damage. In the absence of evidence of its effectiveness, psychotherapy remains a highly experimental procedure that can not justify its preference for its highly decentralized organizational form nor the public's continuing faith in the civic utility of its self-governance.

Without a true clinical role, psychotherapy as a political partisan, even a religious one, stimulates an interpretation of its scholarship as evocative, polemical, and artistic rather than objective. Yet, in contrast with art and polemics, psychotherapy promises concrete measurable outcomes in resolving personal and social problems. These specific, goal-oriented functions—prevention, cure, and rehabilitation—define the principal communal distinction between psychotherapists and artists: the avowed commitment of psychotherapy's practitioners and researchers to decisive objective tests of whether they have reached their goals. While the substance of psychotherapy involves the most deeply subjective human experiences, its claims to professional standing rest on the quality of scientific proofs that its techniques are effective, that they cure, prevent, and rehabilitate.[5]

The conflict between an obligation to objective science and an accommodation with power has dominated the institutional and intellectual development of psychotherapy. This conflict between science and subjectivity helps unravel the paradox of psychotherapy's persistence in spite of its failure to produce any credible evidence of its effectiveness.

The social utility of the field—its value in reaffirming reigning social preferences, its "isomorphism with cultural values"—is independent of its clinical effectiveness.[6] The appearance of its effectiveness and popular belief in its social efficiency are probably sufficient to guarantee the health of the field. The need to appear effective, as distinct from the need to actually be effective, sets the base for the field's mythic function—the creation of metaphors to foster individual adaptation with dominant values, that is, social efficiency. Indeed, psychotherapy's success as political art obscures its deficiencies in the clinic.

The Effectiveness of Psychotherapy: Introversion and Social Narcissism

Personal affirmation, perhaps the vehicle for placebo effects, may be the psychic balm of the therapeutic act. Yet personal affirmation delivered in small doses over a relatively short period of time may be incapable of changing the serious deviant behaviors that are at the core of most psychiatric and social problems: criminality, psychosis, addiction, violence, abuse, neglect, cruelty, and so forth. The thoroughgoing inability of the field to proffer any credible evidence of its effectiveness certainly supports this conclusion.

Psychotherapy may restoreth the soul of only relatively well adjusted people, mild neurotics. Therapists seem to prefer patients who are relatively healthy and successful and whose life experiences are similar to the therapist's.

> The therapist's prejudice against the sick and unimaginative patient is so pronounced that a professional acronym has been created for the ideal subject. It is the YAVIS syndrome—Young, Attractive, Verbal, Intelligent, Successful. Because of this, one suspects that most psychotherapy may not be a treatment for emotional illness at all. It may instead be a cultural, symbolic ritual of the newly sophisticated middle and upper-middle classes for whom it is a mystical corroboration that one is indeed a YAVIS. (Gross 1978, 49–50)

However, there may be a price for emotional compatibility: affirmation junkies who are addicted to therapy and who compulsively seek justification for their self-absorption. In buttressing the self-indulgences of relatively healthy patients who are wealthy enough to afford therapy, the psychotherapeutic process may actually prolong these patients' problems. Affirmation may tend to support the patients' noxious behaviors, allowing them to resist the salutary abrasions of natural social interaction.

The belief in each individual's creativity lies at the core of psychotherapeutic theory, an assumption of spiritual worth that therapy actually holds as a concrete, marketable proposition. However, therapy has no more been able to demonstrate its ability to unlock a patient's suppressed creativity than to reduce frankly deviant behavior. The promise to unleash creativity applied to wealthy, healthy patients as if they were nascent Picassos, Tolstois, and Einsteins reinforces the "secondary gains" of neurosis. It also sounds suspiciously like the confidence game of quacks and charlatans who prey on the lonely, the unhappy, and the unsuccessful. Yet the broader implications of this creed of uniqueness feeds into the culture's preference for an ethic of personal responsibility that displaces a broader social obligation for individual behaviors.

Without a commitment to empiricism, psychotherapy's self-certifying humanism, which in the end may not be at all that humane, corrupts the tests of its effectiveness—the dramas of social myth—through cultlike group processes of thought to conform with its institutional needs. The field's many research weaknesses—expectancy biases, porous measures, convenience sampling, and the rest—are expressions of its cultish demand for unquestioning belief. With the transcendental smugness of the elect, the field dismisses disconfirming evidence, rare as it is, as unusual (e.g., a predictable sampling error), trivial, or in the final step, inconvenient and therefore, invisible.

This epicurean selective perception underscores social self-centeredness, the expectation that psychic adjustment can be purchased as a vanity item of social success. The sacrament of unleashing one's creativity through the incantations of a psychic priest underscores social success as a wonderment of individual motivation that is divorced from any social backdrop of supportive institutions (family, school, and community).

The budget implications are profound. Personal responsibility based upon an immanent theory of psychological functioning entails far fewer public commitments for education, jobs, and family support, as three examples, than a theory that locates personal responsibility in the context of public obligations for supportive social institutions.

The contemporary practice of psychotherapy has become a distorted vulgarization of the intents of its architects, notably Freud, to identify the relationship between the healthy personality and the good society. Adorno's application of Freudian theory to the institutions of a democratic state specifically attempted to work out this relationship for modern culture (Adorno et al. 1969); many other psychoanalysts have also come out from behind their couches to attempt this task (Kurzweil 1989). Despite the many shortcomings of his theories, Freudian psychology represented a belief in the "liberating power of science and reason," applied in the body of Freud's work to a search through the footprints of ancient civilizations for a secular liberal culture that nurtured the human psyche (Schorske 1993). His search for the basis of psychological functioning in social conditions was motivated by a deep personal concern over the institutions of the modern state:

> For no social group did this have more decisive meaning than for the newly emancipated Jews. Their children could join their Christian schoolfellows in acquiring a common gentile culture, the religion of which was...no threat to their own. (Schorske 1993, 35)

In the backwash of the Second World War, Naziism, totalitarianism, and the Holocaust, Adorno and his colleagues attempted to identify the sociological determinants of the prodemocratic personality, thereby relating psychological experience to political outcomes. Attempting a rational approach—a blend of early social psychology, survey technology, and Freudian theory—Adorno and his associates (1969) traced antidemocratic thought and the authoritarian personality back into failed social institutions, notably authoritarian family experiences.

Their specific research task was to define a series of antidemocratic experiences that nurtured psychological intolerance and its realization in the political and social institutions of fascism. Yet their broader purpose, largely fulfilled in Freudian terms of depth psychology, was to identify the experiences that needed to be fostered by the institutions of a democratic state. By implication, these prodemocratic experiences would become the pillars of its humane social policy.

Contemporary psychotherapy has lost this noble civic mission; instead it has come to fulfill a sectarian entrepreneurial role reflecting the preferences of dominant social groups. Consistent with this role, psychotherapy has naturally emerged as the nuclear technique of the private, nonprofit agency sector which is largely the philanthropic arm of commercial and professional elites. These agencies function as powerful ideological voices in addition to their peripheral service roles, replaying the fables of American morality in their choice of service recipients, services, and organizational form.

The psychotherapeutic community has resolved for itself the main conflicts of political and social life. It has rejected a role in justifying a common right to pursue individual identity, values, and position in a "culturally and politically divided modern society." Instead, the psychotherapeutic community has chosen to compose myths of social efficiency and to promulgate them through an institutional attachment to an ethos of clinically based personal adaptation. This is a political choice that expresses the dominant culture's preference for socially efficient service strategies.

The introversion of its social mission—a professional narcissism that is conveniently blind to the social basis of psychological dysfunction—has occurred without any rational support for its clinical effectiveness. Psychotherapy has flourished in spite of its failure as science because its myths satisfy the credo of the culture and the interests of dominant, successful factions.

In a perversion of individuality and personal effort, psychotherapeutic ideology has come to embrace an imagined property of personal creativity and innovation that is to be reclaimed through a personal search for meaning and not a measurable social contribution. Yet in the end, the therapeutic process may recommend little more than a chain hotel personality to conform with an insipid vision of culture—prepackaged, standardized, tasteless, and intolerant.

The Alternatives to Social Efficiency

The myth of social efficiency blocks consideration of alternative solutions for social problems, notably greater investment in the social institutions that are prerequisites for successful participation in contemporary American culture. The costs to achieve an essential or basic level of equality are staggering, multiples of the current federal budget deficit, for filling even simple unmet needs in the United States: assuring every child a special relationship with at least one responsible adult, a high school diploma for all those capable of this level of education, vocational training, jobs, health care, safe sewers and water, secure communities, an adequate retirement, long-term health and mental health care. More intensive services to provide true cultural parity—enriched day care and public education, community services to enhance social and political participation, opportunities for the arts, income supplements to eliminate poverty, environmental protection and preservation, adequate housing, and so forth—are simply beyond any consideration. Yet all of these services may be necessary to realize the civic expectations of a humane modern culture. However, these services cannot be pursued as long as the nation is convinced that current provisions are somehow sufficient, effective, and points of progress in realizing an enlightened American destiny.

In this sense the myth of social efficiency and the subcommunities that sustain it are both socially destructive. By constantly accommodating to the resource limitations of society while claiming ever greater efficiencies in achieving goals, the psychotherapeutic myth condones the abandonment of people in need. From lengthy psychoanalysis, to psychotherapy, to short-term interventions, and now, by turning over its clinical responsibilities to the mercies of market-driven insurance companies, the field has consistently protected its pocketbook and prestige even at the expense of its avowed role in protecting troubled people.

The myth of social efficiency is vulnerable on its central tenet that prior deprivation—deep social inequality—can be redressed cheaply and efficiently. However, social efficiency has not been demonstrated in either the psychotherapeutic literature nor in the larger body of the social service literature. Social problems seem to emerge in some sort of direct relationship to deprivations of basic social institutions: family, community, employment, education. These problems seem to persist in the face of the typically weak interventions of psychotherapy and the social services.

With growing competition over scarce resources, the idea of social efficiency is even more valuable for those with stakes in the current distribution of resources. America's privileged and successful classes indulge the vain arguments that justify their wealth and social position as evidence of their superior character.

Yet, a condition of scarce resources and insatiable appetites constitutes the customary state of society either at impoverished levels or at the levels of American wealth. There is no inherent reason for denying greater social equality. The huge federal deficit in the United States is only the latest state of emergency that contributed to national perceptions of an inability to address deep social problems. Previously wars, inflations and depressions, environmental concerns, consumerism, feminism, the gap in science, industrial productivity, and so forth provided insulation from threatening social claims. These recurrent, near-perpetual crises may be exacerbated in the future by both increasing international competition as well as by the changing demographics of the United States, notably the aging of its population. Only great economic growth or live threats to social stability seem capable of producing a tolerance for a social dividend or broader sharing. However, economic growth at the level of the 1960s is a more unlikely prospect than social turmoil for the United States.

The notion of psychotherapy persists because alternatives to social efficiency are far less politically palatable. If the myth of social efficiency failed as social ideology, implying that psychotherapeutic interventions became politically useless when their ineffectiveness became broadly recognized, then two basic alternative strategies would have to be considered: neglect and greater social equality. Neglect is repugnant and strategies of social equality are vastly more expensive than current social welfare arrangements. Greater public expenditures—for family restoration and preservation, for education, for job creation, training and retraining, for welfare payments, for mental and physical health programs, for long-term care, for housing, and so on—in pursuit of greater social equality are patently not feasible in the contemporary political climate. For the past twenty years the United States has been embarked upon a process of restricting the conditions of citizenship for poorer populations by retrenching its commitment to public services generally.

This retrenchment is likely to continue as an increasingly large proportion of the population ages out of the work force. The demographic changes in the American population over the next thirty years or so and the inability of the American economy to sustain benefits for future retirees at current levels will forcibly reopen the social contract. The enormous pressures for future public obligations in addition to the vast unmet needs of the present American population may impose the fractious myths of social efficiency—that deep social problems can be resolved inexpensively—on a generation's deliberations.

A Final Note: Psychotherapy and the Climate of Contemporary Politics

Political competition over resources has been intensifying in the United States for at least twenty years. While the median income of U.S. families has been stable since 1973, social needs and other claims on the public purse have been increasing.[7] Crime, poverty, unemployment, substance abuse, family dissolution, homelessness, and mental disease have become enormous problems in the United States.

Just a few social indicators capture the gravity of declining social conditions in the United States. Poverty has been increasing for the past few decades. In 1992, the United States added another one million people to its poor, totaling about 15 percent of the entire population, up from a low of 11.1 in 1973 (Committee on Ways and Means 1993, 1313). Moreover, the poverty line is very low in the United States, a bit over fourteen thousand dollars for a family of four in 1992. A true poverty line would probably separate out 25 percent of the population. Thirty-seven million Americans have no health coverage, while health care reform in mid-1994 still seems uncertain. Perhaps as many as one-half million Americans are homeless (Committee on Ways and Means 1993, 1233). Moreover, the United States

> loses one fifth of its children from school in their high school years. The number of candidates for advanced degrees in its universities is declining. Homicide rates per capita are five times the worst found in other industrial countries. The U. S. crowds more than a million convicts into its prisons, among them 40 times as many black prisoners, proportionately, as South Africa at the peak of apartheid. It holds family incomes at mid-1970 levels, even as the average compensation of the managers of failing industrial enterprises ascends from 40 to 90 times their payroll averages. (Piel 1993, 117)

In addition to growing social problems, changes in the marketplace and the family have also increased pressures on public spending. The economic conditions of perhaps half of Americans are perilous. The number of blue collar jobs that pay a wage adequate to support a family has declined while economic safety net programs, notably Aid to Families with Dependent Children (AFDC), have fallen far behind inflation.[8] The decline of a livable wage for many Americans, together with the absence of viable public services and subsidies for families with young children, have forced both spouses in a large number of families to work.

In order to supplement the incomes of their spouses, many parents, particularly mothers, reluctantly increase the amount that they work at the expense of their domestic obligations, notably to their children. The obligation to substitute work for domesticity has increased demands for publicly financed day care and for other services that have been traditionally provided voluntarily by parents. The failure to provide services that compensate for the absence of parents—and the substitution of meager, standardized care, when it is provided at all, for the personalized attention of parents—reduces the social benefits of good homes. Unsupervised children do not bring themselves up well. Inadequate families feed many social problems, notably juvenile delinquency, truancy, poor school performance, and substance abuse.[9]

Life is more threadbare for single parents and their children. One in five American children, frequently living with only one parent, are brought up in poverty. The awful material needs of these children also imply deep cultural deprivations. By and large, children whose families lack adequate resources also frequently lack appropriate supervision, relations with responsible adults, education, and life chances generally. Because the poverty line in the United States is set at arbitrarily low levels, many more families than the officially enumerated poor are living in terrible conditions.

It is deeply troubling for the prospects of a democratic and humane society that the wealthiest nation in the history of the world refuses to extend its bounty to a large portion of its own citizens. No natural barrier prevents Americans from allocating more of their private income to public purposes. Nevertheless, in the face of increasing social distress, Americans in mid-1994 seem very reluctant to increase the very meager categorical benefits of the welfare state, to extend them to the many who need them, and to make the efforts to socialize excluded populations into the mainstream culture.[10]

The refusal to address American social problems with increased resources expresses contemporary American society's pervasive antipathy toward public remedies, signaling the political and ideological ascendancy of economically successful groups. Current social arrangements—the American welfare state and its programs—are deeply entrenched.[11] They are also grossly inadequate, which unfortunately may explain their popularity. In denial of a generous civic culture, the American welfare state has been marching away from the goals of the Enlightenment enterprise for at least two decades. The emotional impetus behind American political choices—a fervor for social efficiency—profoundly rejects greater equality as a solution to its social problems.

Social needs compete for resources and attention against the immense range of factional interests that define contemporary society—defense and foreign affairs, farm subsidies, student grants and loans, research and development, recreation, conservation, and so forth. Indeed, virtually every sector of American society generates claims on the public treasury. Although this conflict over scarce resources is specifically played out over federal budgetary decisions, particularly in reference to the deficit and national debt during recent years, it permeates social discourse generally; after all, budget priorities tend to reflect broader social priorities. Political dialectics to define those priorities seek to justify factional claims in terms of the general good. The immensely complicated script of that justification covers all the corners of social life.

Success in social dialectics can have powerful consequences, justifying the extent to which private resources are converted into particular public purposes through taxes and the extent to which particular groups are rewarded with those resources for performing tasks in the society's interests. Because private preferences tend to be congruent with public purposes, victors in the competition over the public budget also tend to receive the society's unmandated rewards of prestige and access.

The field of psychotherapy, by failing to objectively assess its effectiveness and by mystifying its clinical interventions as scientific knowledge, participates in contemporary social dialectics on behalf of dominant political interests. Popular antagonisms toward a public policy of greater equality find expression in the psychotherapy literature as a series of relatively inexpensive and superficial treatments. Furthermore, the field's insistence upon its clinical effectiveness—the success of its interventions in reforming deviant behaviors that are at the heart of social problems—cements the culture's sublime attachment to a bald ethic of personal responsibility while minimizing any deeper obligation for greater investments in individual performance. The belief in the patient's ability to change his or her behavior through a brief course of self-exploration or self-control is at the core of psychotherapy. This reliance upon an inspired will as the source of therapeutic change is argued through the field's outcome studies. However, these chapters in the pseudoscience of psychotherapy, even dressed in the robes of science, fail to distinguish psychotherapeutic interventions from the exhortations of tent revivals, missionaries, and twelve-step self-help groups. Just as resistance to the wafer invites eternal damnation and communal scorn, the patient's failure to accept the secular epiphany of psychotherapy signals a flaw of character that quietly exonerates a neglectful public policy from more intensive and expensive attempts at reform.

Psychotherapy's production of misleading support for its social efficiency is also political evidence that more extensive strategies to handle social problems are not necessary. However, in conniving for political congeniality, the field has lost standing for scientific probity. The refusal of the psychotherapeutic subcommunity to acknowledge its scholarly deficiencies, its apparent ineffectiveness, and its possible harm are more than the innocent adolescent peccadillos of an emerging field. Psychotherapeutic research has been around for decades and, with the broad social sanction implied by government funding, it is conducted in knowing defiance of rigorous scientific standards.

The absence of a credible clinical role underscores the ideological role that psychotherapy plays in social dialects. The notion of social efficiency captures its essential ideological utility, placing psychotherapeutics and social therapies generally at the heart of the conflict over scarce resources. In the context of heated political competition, psychotherapy is an attractive justification that denies greater resources to a variety of social claims. If inexpensive talking—moral suasion of one sort or another—fails, then social problems require more thoroughgoing solutions commanding the expenditure of additional moneys with all of its unpleasant implications for the redistribution of income and wealth through taxation to fund increased government services.

If the culture is to resolve its social problems then it needs to confront the reality implied by the failure of psychotherapy's minimal interventions: more is needed to resolve social need. However, current enthusiasms for postmodern methods of thought in the social sciences and in the culture generally create precisely the wrong mood for a confrontation with the realities of American neglect.

The postmodern analysis of contemporary society characteristically employs subjective and idiosyncratic methods for establishing truth. Its common "methods of deconstruction and intuitive interpretation" recall other more traditional lapses in proof that reject an objective reality in favor of experiential wisdom, magic, mystery, phenomenology, hermeneutics, the occult, and spectral proofs (Rosenau 1992, 23).

> Post-modern methodology is post-positivist or anti-positivist. As substitutes for the "scientific method," the [affirmative post-modernists] look to feelings, personal experience, empathy, emotion, intuition, subjective judgment, imagination, as well as diverse forms of creativity and play. But the actual content of these terms and their methodological significance are relatively vague and difficult to communicate to others. The skeptical post-modernists might deny most of these as substitutes for method because, they argue, we can never really know anything, not even our own feelings and emotions. (Rosenau 1992, 117–118)

Postmodernism strengthens the social mood that diminishes rational processes and objective proofs. Its more "practical" methods better satisfy the discursive requirements of partisans. In this sense, postmodernism is construed more broadly than simply a particular school of analysis that rejects objective rationality. Postmodernism emphasizes the subjective not simply as an important element in personal meaning, but as the central construct in defining, interpreting, and evaluating society.

Postmodernism is an expression of antirational, philosophic nihilism that denies the possibility of any authority, notably science and religion, whose source of legitimacy is located outside of society. In its most powerful form, the postmodern critique argues that central cultural values, unbounded by any consideration for justice, decency, rationality or fairness, perfuse all social decision making. The critique has pointed to the depravities of socialist and capitalist regimes alike and to the inability of the modern liberal state to correct those failures. Yet, while the postmodern critique rejects the political forms inspired by the Enlightenment—capitalism, socialism, and the modern liberal state—it fails to define an alternative to its thicket of subjectivity. Paradoxically, its rejection of modernity, following the logic of its interpretive "proofs," has undermined its own sympathies for the powerless and the socially marginal. For, as a philosophy of despair and lost purpose, postmodernism

> has now passed over into a species of disguised apologetics for the socio-political status quo, a persuasion that "reality" is constituted through and through by the meanings, values or discourses that presently compose it, so that nothing could count as effective counterargument, much less a critique of existing institutions on valid theoretical grounds. (Norris 1990, 3-4)

Even the best postmodern arguments, in a fervor to transcend the limits of social reality, more often than not produce ahistorical and whimsical treatments of social problems. It is not coincidental that deconstructionism and other postmodern analyses parallel the rise of the religious right; the resurgence of mind and body cures; the growth of mysticism, healing cults, and "alternative medical therapies"; and the renewal of the case against science. Postmodern ideologies, techniques, and assumptions feed into ferocious needs for ennoblement and self-affirmation and, therefore, lead to a reliance upon revealed authority, unquestioning belief, faith, and self-certification. Indeed, postmodernism itself may be understood as a fearful reaction to the gloomy failures of the modern era.

The challenge of the postmodern critique to rational discourse stems out of its emphasis upon a social construction of reality, a nice literary device but in its broad use as an explanatory tool, one that carries along the liability of arbitrary causality. The plausibility of a socially constructed reality has lead to the fallacy, a frequent conceit of the intellectual, that society is only the product of human wishes (i.e., ideology). In this way, political, social, and economic events appear as easy consequences of an improved discourse, that is, a newly contrived social will or consciousness.

In spite of their superficial commitments to science, psychotherapy and social therapeutics generally are animated by postmodern subjectivities even while they have both become objects of postmodern criticism. Yet, by practicing the subjective parody of rigorous science, psychotherapy creates a sham of service. Embellished and dramatized through clinical practice, psychotherapeutic myths play a powerful role in the narrative that subordinates the claims of those in need to the dominant political interests that thrive on current social inequities.

The failure of psychotherapy as a credible clinical intervention and its success as ideology stand as witnesses for the broad postmodern critique of the Enlightenment enterprise, particularly the implausibility of scientific neutrality in pursuit of a humane social policy. Nevertheless, the apparent relevance of the postmodern critique to psychotherapy as a pawn of the dominant social ethos does not by itself condemn the value of scientific objectivity in pursuit of truth, rationality, and social progress. Even more importantly, the miscarriage of a particular scientific undertaking such as psychotherapy does not justify greater subjectivity in assessing the conditions of society.

The current mood of politics proved irresistible for psychotherapy. The competition over scarce resources created an appetite for postmodern scientism that psychotherapy is satisfying. However, in creating the illusions of a comforting social reality, the field of psychotherapy has capitulated to the sublime forces of culture and destroyed the credibility of its own counsel. The deplorable shape of the psychotherapeutic literature is a cautionary wreck of what happens when objective science and decency are sacrificed to political compatibility and professional success.

Notes

1. Critics are too easily dismissed. As one common example, Lambert and Bergin (in Bergin and Garfield 1994) handle the Prioleau et al. (1983) concern with placebo effects on largely consensual grounds:

   > The most controversial article on this subject was published by Prioleau et al. (1983).... Prioleau et al. interpreted these data as suggesting that formal psychotherapy was not more effective than placebo therapies designed to emphasize attention and support, but the validity of the conclusion of this review were seriously questioned in the majority of commentaries accompanying the article. Prioleau et al.'s conclusions cannot be accepted at face value. (150)

   Their conclusion is more appropriately applied to the body of psychotherapy's outcome research than to Prioleau et al.
2. The idea of the cult is not simply a neutral descriptor of an emerging and novel minority thought system. The characteristics of a cult are antithetical to the personal traits and group processes that are cherished by a scientific community and by its supportive civic culture. Cults, in contrast with scientific communities, impose a group personality in place of individuality; the narrow organizational needs of the group over individual development; revelation and doctrinal truths as substitutes for objective truths; indisputable, often charismatic, authority instead of protected skepticism and dissent. Psychotherapy has many of the characteristics of an enveloping religion, walled off in communities of believers by dogma and true belief from empirical verification of its value. Its internal pro-

cesses of communication recall those of religious cults more than scientific subcommunities.

The characteristics of psychotherapists may often coincide with Bainbridges' (1978) criteria for the cultish personality. Gross (1978) presented evidence that as many as 75 percent of psychotherapists have been and continue to be in therapy or analysis, suggesting that they have experienced "acutely felt tensions." It also seems reasonable that the calling to the heroic role of psychic healer—a "seekership"—is most frequently, if not always, a result of personal distress. Gross also convincingly reinterprets psychotherapy as a religion, employing emotional rather than rational problem-solving techniques. Graduate education is frequently a "turning point" that provides "affective bonds" and "intensive interaction" within the community of therapists. Therapists may also be a very separate and self-reliant group with relatively few attachments outside of their own little band of prophets.

Psychotherapy researchers may go through a similar socialization. Instead of independent investigators who are drawn to the intellectual problems of the field, they may also be cultic converts who have been resurrected from their psychic distress through therapy. In fact, the epiphanies of the researchers may be particularly intense. As the myth makers of therapy, they may need to believe more completely in the power of therapy than practitioners or patients in order to translate between professional ambitions and social convenience and to justify continuing investments in psychotherapeutic practice on grounds of its effectiveness and social utility.

It is difficult to assess the intensity of the group experience for the members of the psychotherapeutic subcommunity. Yet its many cultish tendencies establish ostensible grounds on which to understand the near-uniform absence of credible tests of its outcomes and a pervasive hostility to independent scrutiny. The polite summary of professional psychotherapy as an intense group experience looses the essentially coercive nature of its group thought—the insistence upon conformity, fervor of belief, and central control conveyed by the idea of a cult. Sheltered from demands for objective accountability, psychotherapy has created its own ideology of humanism—subjective and untested mythological systems of interpretation and complex catechisms of temptations, sins, and virtues.

Psychotherapy is not yet a cult in the sense of Scientology. Quite to the contrary, it is a mainstream thought system that sits at the very core of established cultural beliefs. Yet, many groups on the periphery of psychotherapy are clearly cults (e.g., Mari-el therapists, past life healers, EST, many portions of the self-help movement, a number of therapeutic communities for treating substance abuse), drawing their own therapeutic insights from mainline doctrine and proof in the same manner that Christian cults rely upon their own idiosyncratic interpretations of Christian texts and practices. Nevertheless, the scientific standing of mainstream psychotherapy is no different from that of its own cults, while the psychotherapeutic community's methods for testing the truth of its propositions and the effectiveness of its interventions accepts an essentially cultlike group process of self-certification.

Psychotherapy has created a cultic milieu that derives its specialness not from its cultural deviance—psychotherapy is a central cultural institution—but from its sense of the unknowable, the mystical, the hidden, and its rare powers of healing. The psychotherapy subcommunity has organized itself as though it were a restricted club of spiritual alchemists who magically dispel psychic distress with hidden powers.

The true heterodoxy of psychotherapy lies in its sublime subjectivity, its employment of unorthodox science. The cultic tendencies of psychotherapy are bound together by its attractiveness to a credulous public seeking psychic release; "seekership is probably the one characteristic that all members of cultic groups have in common" (Campbell 1972, 127). The seekership of psychotherapy is greatly facilitated by its weak scholarship, a bogus science, that produces consistently false but high-status testimonials to its curative abilities.

3. Pallone (1988) even suggests that psychotherapy's main function is to create and punish bad examples of personal behavior: "we fulfill roles vital to the maintenance of a society in which visible, publicly identifiable deviance is a necessity" (69).
4. The role of a cultish fundamentalism in supporting the New Right in the United States would seem to belie this artificial and perhaps naive separation of the religious and the political in considering social ideology.
5. It is important to distinguish the source of an inspiration from the fact of its clinical effectiveness. Whatever the broader merits of a particular proposition—its influence in leading to valuable insights, or the nature of its discovery—its clinical value is established by rigorous scientific testing. In this light, Thomas Nagel (1994) argues that Freud's contribution as philosopher, social critic, and visionary transcends the scientific meaning of psychoanalysis, its clinical effectiveness. Well and good, there are different criteria for different uses. But Nagel's defense of Freud the thinker is *not* a defense of the clinical value of psychoanalysis.
6. Meyer and Rowan (1977) suggested that organizations fall along a single continuum running from "isomorphism with cultural values" to a true production function. However, these are two separate dimensions and organizations exhibit different degrees of both. Yet, their notion of a political function in organizations is very helpful in trying to explain the persistence of organizations that do not seem to provide any direct service or product and organizations that do not seem to be constrained by their apparent goals.
7. Per capita family income as reported in Bureau of the Census 1991, table B-4 and current social needs as detailed throughout the Green Book (Committee on Ways and Means 1993).
8. In constant 1992 dollars average payments per person on AFDC have fallen from $166 in 1970 to $136 in 1992 (Committee on Ways and Means 1993, 668.)
9. The GNP as a measure of the *social good* might be discounted by the degree to which socially beneficial behaviors such as parenting are diminished by economically valuable behaviors such as the provision of work. In this sense, economic growth is not an adequate measure of social welfare unless it includes all of the goods and services that a society requires and not simply those that are provided in commercial markets.
10. Even the present administration's very modest proposals for welfare reform in mid-1994 seem to be in peril.
11. Cook and Barrett (1992) take heart from occasionally sizable public opinions to increase the benefits of a number of welfare programs. However, their survey probably reflected a large amount of stereotypical "goodness" as respondents may have frequently reported what they thought was expected of them more than their true feelings. For example, the reported priorities of both Congressional respondents and public respondents favored poor children. Yet, the legislative inactivity on their behalf is probably a truer indicator of the national mood than the reported opinions of respondents.

References

Abramowitz, S. I. and N. W. Bell. 1985. "Biofeedback, Self-Control and Tension Headache." *Journal of Psychosomatic Research* 29(1): 95-99.

Adams, J. F., F. P. Piercey, and J. A. Jurich. 1991. "Effects of Solution Focused Therapy's 'Formula First Session Task' on Compliance and Outcome in Family Therapy." *Journal of Marital and Family Therapy* 17(3): 277-90.

Adorno, T. W., E. Frenkel-Brunswik, D. J. Levinson, and R. N. Sanford. 1969 (originally published 1950). *The Authoritarian Personality*. New York: W. W. Norton.

Alden, L. 1989. "Short-Term Structured Treatment for Avoidant Personality Disorder." *Journal of Consulting and Clinical Psychology* 57(6): 756-64.

Alexander, P. C., R. A. Neimeyer, V. M. Follette, M. K. Moore, and S. Harter. 1989. "A Comparison of Group Treatments of Women Sexually Abused as Children." *Journal of Consulting and Clinical Psychology* 57(4): 479-83.

American Psychiatric Association. 1989. *Treatments of Psychiatric Disorders: A Task Force Report of the American Psychiatric Association*. Washington, D.C.: American Psychiatric Association.

Andrews, D. A., I. Zinger, R. D. Hoge, J. Bonta, P. Gendreau, and F. T. Cullen. 1990. "Does Correctional Treatment Work? A Clinically Relevant and Psychologically Informed Meta-analysis." *Criminology* 28(3): 419-29.

Andrews, G. and R. Harvey. 1981. "Does Psychotherapy Benefit Neurotic Patients." *Archives of General Psychiatry* 38(November): 1203-08.

Appleyard, B. 1992. *Understanding the Present*. New York: Doubleday.

Azrin, N. H., V. A. Besalel, R. Bechtel, A. Michalicek, M. Mancera, D. Carroll, D. Shuford, and J. Cox. 1980. "Comparison of Reciprocity and Discussion-Type Counseling for Marital Problems." *American Journal of Family Therapy* 8: 21-28.

Bagarozzi, D. A. and P. Rauen. 1981. "Premarital Counseling: Appraisal and Status." *American Journal of Family Therapy* 9(3): 13-30.

Baggs, K. and S. H. Spence. 1990. "Effectiveness of Booster Sessions in the Maintenance and Enhancement of Treatment Gains Following Assertion Training." *Journal of Consulting and Clinical Psychology* 58(6): 845-54.

Bainbridge, W. S. 1978. *Satan's Power*. Berkeley: University of California Press.

Barkley, R. A., D. C. Guevremont, A. D. Anastopoulos, and K. E. Fletcher. 1992. "A Comparison of Three Family Therapy Programs for Treating Family Conflicts in Adolescents with Attention-Deficit Hyperactivity Disorder." *Journal of Consulting and Clinical Psychology* 60(3): 450-62.

Barlow, D. H., G. T. O'Brien, and C. G. Last. 1984. "Couples Treatment of Agoraphobia." *Behavior Therapy* 15: 41-58.

Baucom, D. H., S. L. Sayers, and T. G. Sher. 1990. "Supplementing Behavioral Marital Therapy with Cognitive Restructuring and Emotional Expressiveness Training: An Outcome Investigation." *Journal of Consulting and Clinical Psychology* 58(5): 636-45.

Baucom, D. H. and G. W. Lester. 1986. "The Usefulness of Cognitive Restructuring as an Adjunct to Behavioral Marital Therapy." *Behavior Therapy* 17: 385–403.

Beach, S. R. H. and K. D. O'Leary. 1986. "The Treatment of Depression Occurring in the Context of Marital Discord." *Behavior Therapy* 17: 43–49.

Beck, D. F. 1975. "Research Findings on the Outcomes of Marital Counseling." *Social Casework* (March): 153–82.

Becker, E. 1973. *Denial of Death*. New York: Free Press.

Behrens, B. C., M. R. Sanders, and W. K. Halford. 1990. "Behavioral Marital Therapy: An Evaluation of Treatment Effects Across High and Low Risk Settings." *Behavior Therapy* 21: 423–33.

Bellack, A. S., M. Hersen, and J. Himmelhoch. 1981. "Social Skills Training Compared with Pharmacotherapy and Psychotherapy in the Treatment of Unipolar Depression." *American Journal of Psychiatry* 138(12 December): 1562–67.

Berger, L. S. 1991. *Substance Abuse as Symptom*. Hillsdale, N.J.: The Analytic Press.

Bergin, A. E. 1971. "The Evaluation of Therapeutic Outcomes." S. L. Garfield and A. E. Begin (eds.). *Handbook of Psychotherapy and Behavior Change*. New York: John Wiley.

———. 1975. "Individual Psychotherapy and Behavior Therapy." *Annual Review of Psychotherapy and Behavior Therapy* 26: 509–56.

———. 1980. "Negative Effects Revisited: A Reply." *Professional Psychology*. (February): 93–100.

Bergin, A. E. and M. J. Lambert. 1978. "The Evaluation of Therapeutic Outcomes." S. L. Garfield and A. E. Bergin (eds.). *Handbook of Psychotherapy and Behavior Change*. New York: John Wiley.

Bergin, A. E. and S. L. Garfield (eds.). *Handbook of Psychotherapy and Behavior Change*. New York: John Wiley.

Berlin, I. 1981. *Personal Impressions*. Middelesex: Penguin Books.

Berman, J. S., R. C. Miller, and P. J. Massman. 1985. "Cognitive Therapy Versus Systematic Desensitization: Is One Treatment Superior?" *Psychological Bulletin* 97(3): 451–61.

Blanchard, E. B., F. Andrasik, T. A. Ahles, S. J. Teders, and D. O'Keefe. 1980. "Migraine and Tension Headache: A Meta-Analytic Review." *Behavior Therapy* 11: 613–31.

Blanchard, E. B. and F. Andrasik. 1982. "Psychological Assessment and Treatment of Headache: Recent Developments and Emerging Issues." *Journal of Consulting and Clinical Psychology* 50(6): 859–79.

Bland, K. and R. S. Hallam. 1981. "Relationship Between Response to Graded Exposure and Marital Satisfaction in Agoraphobics." *Behavioral Research and Therapy* 19: 335–38.

Boelens, W., P. Emmelkamp, D. MacGilla, and M. Markvoor. 1980. "A Clinical Evaluation of Marital Treatment: Reciprocity Counseling vs. System-Theoretic Counseling." *Behavioral Analysis and Modification* 4: 85–96.

Bond, G. R., E. C. McDonel, L. D. Miller, and M. Pensec. 1991. "Assertive Community Treatment and Reference Groups: An Evaluation of Their Effectiveness for Young Adults with Serious Mental Illness and Substance Abuse Problems." *Psychosocial Rehabilitation Journal* 15(2): 31–43.

Borkovec, T. D. 1982. "Insomnia." *Journal of Consulting and Clinical Psychology* 50(6): 880–95.

Botvin, G. J., E. Baker, L. Dusenbury, S. Tortu, and E. M. Botvin. 1990. "Preventing Adolescent Drug Abuse Through a Multimodal Cognitive-Behavioral Approach:

Results of a 3-Year Study." *Journal of Consulting and Clinical Psychology* 58(4): 437-46.

Bowers, T. G. and M. R. Al-Redha. 1990. "A Comparison of Outcome with Group/Marital and Standard/Individual Therapies with Alcoholics." *Journal of Studies on Alcohol* 51(4): 301-09.

Brock, G. W. and H. Joanning. 1983. "A Comparison of the Relationship Enhancement Program and the Minnesota Couple Communication Program." *Journal of Marital and Family Therapy* 9(4): 413-21.

Brom, D., R. J. Kleber, and P. B. Defares. 1989. "Brief Psychotherapy for Posttraumatic Stress Disorders." *Journal of Consulting and Clinical Psychology* 57(5): 607-12.

Bureau of the Census, Department of Commerce. 1991. "Money Income of Households, Families, and Persons in the United States: 1990." *Current Population Reports,* series P-60, no. 174.

Burton, M. V., R. W. Parker, and J. M. Wollner. 1991. "The Psychotherapeutic Value of a 'Chat': A Verbal Response Modes Study of a Placebo Attention Control with Breast Cancer Patients." *Psychotherapy Research* 1(1): 39-61.

Butler, G., M. Fennell, P. Robson, and M. Gelder. 1991. "Comparison of Behavior Therapy and Cognitive Behavior Therapy in the Treatment of Generalized Anxiety Disorder." *Journal of Consulting and Clinical Psychology* 59(1): 167-75.

Campbell, C. 1972. "Cult, The Cultic Milieu and Secularization," in *A Sociological Yearbook of Religion in Britain*. London: SCM Press, 119-36.

Carpenter, W. T., D. W. Heinrichs, and T. E. Hanlon. 1987. "A Comparative Trial of Pharmacologic Strategies in Schizophrenia. 139th Annual Meeting of the American Psychiatric Association (1986, Washington, D.C.)." *American Journal of Psychiatry* 144(11): 1466-70.

Carroll, K. M., B. J. Rounsaville, and F. H. Gawin. 1991. "A Comparative Trial of Psychotherapies for Ambulatory Cocaine Abusers: Relapse Prevention and Interpersonal Psychotherapy." *American Journal of Drug and Alcohol Abuse* 17(3): 229-47.

Casey, R. J. and J. S. Berman. 1985. "The Outcome of Psychotherapy with Children." *Psychological Bulletin* 98: 388-400.

Clarke, G., H. Hops, P. M. Lewinsohn, J. Andrews, J. R. Seeley, and J. Williams. 1992. "Cognitive-Behavioral Group Treatment of Adolescent Depression: Prediction of Outcome." *Behavior Therapy* 23: 341-54.

Clarkin, J. F., I. D. Glick, G. L. Haas, J. H. Spencer, A. B. Lewis, J. Peyser, N. DeMane, M. Good-Ellis, E. Harris, and V. Lestelle. 1990. "A Randomized Clinical Trial of Inpatient Family Intervention: V. Results for Affective Disorders." *Journal of Affective Disorders* 18: 17-28.

Cloward, R. and I. Epstein. 1967. "Private Social Welfare's Disengagement from the Poor." In G. Brager and E. Purcel (eds.) *Community Action Against Poverty*. New Haven, Conn.: College and University Press.

Cobb, J. P., A. M. Mathews, C. A. Childs, and C. M. Blowers. 1984. "The Spouse as Co-Therapist in the Treatment of Agoraphobia." *British Journal of Psychiatry* 144: 282-87.

Coleman, D. J. and M. S. Kaplan. 1990. "Effects of Pretherapy Videotape Preparation on Child Therapy Outcomes." *Professional Psychology Research and Practice* 21(3): 199-203.

Committee on Ways and Means, U. S. House of Representatives. 1993. *1993 Green Book: Overview of Entitlement Programs*. Washington, D.C.: U.S. Government Printing Office.

Cook, F. L. and E. J. Barrett. 1992. *Support for the American Welfare State*. New York: Columbia University Press.

Cooper, N. A. and G. A. Clum. 1989. "Imaginal Flooding as a Supplementary Treatment for PTSD in Combat Veterans: A Controlled Study." *Behavior Therapy* 20: 381-91.

Cooper, S. E. 1983. "The Influence of Self-Concept on Outcomes of Intensive Alcoholism Treatment." *Journal of Studies on Alcohol* 44(6): 1087-93.

Crews, F. 1993. "The Unknown Freud." *New York Review* 30(19): 55-66.

Crisp, A. H., K. Norton, S. Gowers, C. Halek, C. Bowyer, D. Yeldham, G. Levitt, and A. Bhat. 1991. "A Controlled Study of the Effect of Therapies Aimed at Adolescent and Family Psychopathology in Anorexia Nervosa." *British Journal of Psychiatry* 159: 325-33.

Cross, D. G., P. W. Sheehan, and J. A. Kahn. 1980. "Alternative Advice and Counsel in Psychotherapy." *Journal of Consulting and Clinical Psychology* 48(5): 615-25.

Dawes, R. M. 1994. *House of Cards: Psychology and Psychotherapy Built on Myth*. New York: The Free Press.

de Carufel, F. L. and W. E. Piper. 1988. "Group Psychotherapy or Individual Psychotherapy: Patient Characteristics as Predictive Factors." *International Journal of Group Psychotherapy* 38(2): 169-88.

DeRubeis, R. J., M. D. Evans, and S. D. Hollon. 1990. "How Does Cognitive Therapy Work? Cognitive Change and Symptom Change in Cognitive Therapy and Pharmacotherapy for Depression." *Journal of Consulting and Clinical Psychology* 58(6): 862-69.

Deutsch, H. 1980. *The Therapeutic Process, the Self, and Female Psychology*. New Brunswick, N.J.: Transaction Publishers.

DeWitt, K. N. 1978. "The Effectiveness of Family Therapy." *Archives of General Psychiatry* 35(May): 549-61.

Druckman, D. and R. A. Bjork (eds.). 1991. *In the Mind's Eye; Enhancing Human Performance*. Washington, D.C.: National Academy Press.

Druckman, D. and A. Swets (eds.). 1988. *Enhancing Human Performance: Issues, Theories, and Techniques*. Washington, D.C.: National Academy Press.

Dryden, W. and Feltham, C. 1992. *Psychotherapy and its Discontents*. Buckingham: Open University Press.

Dush, D., M. L. Hirt, and H. E. Schroeder. 1983. "Self-statement Modification with Adults: A Meta-Analysis." *Psychological Bulletin* 94(3): 408-22.

Eisenberg, D. M., R. C. Kessler, C. Foster, F. E Norlock, D. R. Calkins, and T. L. Delbanco. 1993. "Unconventional Medicine in the United States." *New England Journal of Medicine* 28(January): 246-52.

Elizur, J. and S. Minuchin. 1989. *Institutionalizing Madness*. New York: Basic Books.

Elkin, I., I. T. Shea, J. T. Watkins, S. D. Imber, S. M. Sotsky, J. F. Collins, D. R. Glass, P. A. Pilkonis, W. R. Leber, J. P. Docherty, S. J. Fiester, and M. B. Parloff. 1989. "National Institute of Mental Health Treatment of Depression Collaborative Research Program." *Archives of General Psychiatry* 46(November): 971-83.

Emmelkamp, P. M. G. 1980. "Agoraphobics' Interpersonal Problems." *Archives of General Psychiatry* 37: 1303-06.

Emmelkamp, P. M. G. and I. DeLange. 1983. "Spouse Involvement in the Treatment of Obsessive-Compulsive Patients." *Behavioral Research and Therapy* 21(4): 341-46.

Epstein, L. 1992. (Book review) *The Rise of the Therapeutic State* by A. J. Polsky, *Social Service Review* 66(4): 654-58.

Epstein, W. M. 1984a. "Technology and Social Work 1: The Effectiveness of Psychotherapy." *Journal of Applied Social Sciences* 8(2): 155–75.

———. 1984b. "Technology and Social Work 2: Psychotherapy, Family Therapy and Implications for Practice." *Journal of Applied Social Sciences* 8(2): 175–87.

———. 1993. *The Dilemma of American Social Welfare*. New Brunswick, N.J.: Transaction Publishers.

———. "Economic Development and Social Welfare in the Third World: The End of Romance." *International Journal of Comparative and Social Welfare* (in press).

Eysenck, H. F. 1952. "The Effects of Psychotherapy: An Evaluation." *Journal of Consulting Psychology* 16: 319.

———. 1961. "The Effects of Psychotherapy" in H. F. Eysenck (ed.). *Handbook of Abnormal Psychology*. New York: Basic Books.

———. 1965. "The Effects of Psychotherapy." *International Journal of Psychiatry* 1: 97.

Eysenck, H. F. and Rachman, S. 1965. *Causes and Cures of Neuroses*. London: Routledge and Kegan Paul.

Fairburn, C. G., J. Kirk, M. O'Connor, and P. J. Cooper. 1986. "A Comparison of Two Psychological Treatments for Bulimia Nervosa." *Behaviour Research and Therapy* 24(6): 629–43.

Falloon, F. R. H. 1982. "Family Management in the Prevention of Exacerbations of Schizophrenia." *New England Journal of Medicine* 306(24): 1437–40.

Ferris, T. 1993. (Book review) "The Case Against Science." *Understanding the Present* by B. Appleyard, *New York Review of Books* (May 13): 17–19.

Fettes, P. A. and J. M. Peters. 1992. "A Meta-Analysis of Group Treatments for Bulimia Nervosa." *International Journal of Eating Disorders* 11(2): 97–110.

Figley, C. R. 1989. *Treating Family Stress*. New York: Bruner/Mazel Inc.

Fischer, J. 1973. "Is Casework Effective: A Review." *Social Work* 18(1): 5–20.

Fleischman, M. J. and S. A. Szykula. 1981. "A Community Setting Replication of a Social Learning Treatment for Aggressive Children." *Behavior Therapy* 12: 115–22.

Flowers, J. V. and C. D. Booraem. 1991. "A Psychoeducational Group for Clients with Heterogeneous Problems: Process and Outcomes." *Small Group Research* 22(2): 258–73.

Formiani, R. 1990. *The Myth of Scientific Public Policy*. New Brunswick, N.J.: Transaction Publishers.

Frank, A. F. and J. G. Gunderson. 1990. "The Role of the Therapeutic Alliance in the Treatment of Schizophrenia." *Archives of General Psychiatry* 47(March): 228–36.

Frank, J. D. and J. B. Frank. 1991 (Third Edition). *Persuasion and Healing*. Baltimore: The Johns Hopkins University Press.

Franks, C. M. and D. T. Mays. 1980. "Negative Effects Revisited: A Rejoinder." *Professional Psychology* 11: 101–05.

Freeman, C., F. Sinclair, J. Turnbull, and A. Annandale. 1985. "Psychotherapy for Bulimia: A Controlled Study. Conference on Anorexia Nervosa and Related Disorders (1984, Swansea, Wales)." *Journal of Psychiatric Research* 19(2–3): 473–78.

Friedman, A. S. 1989. "Family Therapy vs. Parent Groups: Effects on Adolescent Drug Abusers." *American Journal of Family Therapy* 17(4): 335–47.

Gardner, M. 1988. "Bumps on the Head" (book review). *Pseudo-science and Society in Nineteenth Century America* by A. Wrobel. *New York Review of Books*.

Garfield, S. L. and A. E. Bergin (eds.). 1971, 1978, 1986. *Handbook of Psychotherapy and Behavior Change*. New York: John Wiley.

Giblin, P., D. H. Sprenkle, and R. Sheehan. 1985. "Enrichment Outcome Research: A Meta-Analysis of Premarital, Marital and Family Interventions." *Journal of Marital and Family Therapy* 11(3): 257–71.

Girodo, M., S. J. Stein, and S. E. Dotzenroth. 1980. "The Effects of Communication Skills Training and Contracting on Marital Relations." *Behavioral Engineering* 6(2): 61–76.

Glaister, B. 1982. "Muscle Relaxation Training for Fear Reduction of Patients with Psychological Problems: A Review of Controlled Studies." *Behavior Research Therapy* 20: 493–504.

Glick, I. D., L. Fleming, N. Dechillo, N. Meyerkop, C. Jackson, D. Muscara, and M. Goodelli. 1986. "A Controlled Study of Transitional Day Care for Non-Chronically-Ill Patients." *American Journal of Psychiatry* 143(12): 1551–56.

Glick, I. D., J. F. Clarkin, J.. H. Spencer, G. L. Haas, A. B. Lewis, J. Peyser, N. Demane, M. Goodelli, E. Harris, and V. Lestelle. 1985. "A Controlled Evaluation of Inpatient Family Intervention: I. Preliminary Results of the Six-Month Follow-Up." *Archives of General Psychiatry* 42(9): 882–86.

Goldberg, R. J. and M. S. Wool. 1985. "Psychotherapy for the Spouses of Lung Cancer Patients: Assessment of an Intervention." *Psychotherapy and Psychosomatics* 43(3): 141–50.

Gross, M. L. 1978. *The Psychological Society*. New York: Random House.

Grunbaum, A. 1984. *The Foundations of Psychoanalysis*. Berkeley: University of California Press.

Gurman, A. S. 1973. "The Effects and Effectiveness of Marital Therapy: A Review of Outcome Research." *Family Process* 12: 145–70.

Gurman, A. S. and D. P. Kniskern. 1977. "Enriching Research on Marital Enrichment Programs." *Journal of Marriage and Family Counseling*, 3: 3–11.

———. 1978a. "Behavioral Marriage Therapy: II. Empirical Perspective." *Family Process* 17: 139–48.

———. 1978b. "Research on Marital and Family Therapy: Progress, Perspective and Prospect," In S. L. Garfield and A. E. Begin (eds.). *Handbook of Psychotherapy and Behavior Change*. New York: John Wiley.

———. 1986. "Research on Marital and Family Therapy: Progress, Perspective, and Prospect." In S. L. Garfield and A. E. Begin (eds.). *Handbook of Psychotherapy and Behavior Change* (2nd ed). New York: John Wiley, 817–902.

Haas, G. L., I. D. Glick, J. F. Clarkin, J. H. Spencer, A. B. Lewis, J. Peyser, N. Demane, M. Goodelli, E. Harris, and V. Lestelle. 1988. "Inpatient Family Intervention: A Randomized Clinical Trial: II. Results at Hospital Discharge." *Archives of General Psychiatry* 45(3): 217–24.

Hafner, R. J., A. Badenoch, J. Fisher, and H. Swift. 1983. "Spouse-Aided Versus Individual Therapy in Persisting Psychiatric Disorders: A Systematic Comparison." *Family Process* 22: 385–99.

Hahlweg, K. 1982. "Treatment of Marital Distress: Comparing Formats and Modalities." *Advances in Behavior Research Therapy* 4: 57–74.

Hahlweg, K. and H. J. Markman. 1988. "Effectiveness of Behavioral Marital Therapy: Empirical Status of Behavioral Techniques in Preventing and Alleviating Marital Distress." *Journal of Consulting and Clinical Psychology* 56(3): 440–47.

Hall, A. and A. H. Crisp. 1987. "Brief Psychotherapy in the Treatment of Anorexia Nervosa: Outcome at One Year." *British Journal of Psychiatry* 151: 185–91.

Hawton, K., S. McKeown, A. Day, P. Martin, M. O'Connor, and S. Yule. 1987. "Evaluation of Out-Patient Counselling Compared with General Practitioner Care Following Overdoses." *Psychological Medicine* 17(3): 751–61.

Heineman Pieper, M. 1989. "The Heuristic Paradigm; A Unifying and Comprehensive Approach to Social Work Research." *Smith College Studies in Social Work* 60(1): 8-34.

Heller, S. 1993. "After Orientalism: Exploring the Complicity of Literature and Empire." *Chronicle of Higher Education* (May 19): A8-A10.

Henggeler, S. W. 1991. "Effects of Multisystemic Therapy on Drug Use and Abuse in Serious Juvenile Offenders: A Progress Report from Two Outcome Studies." *Family Dynamics of Addiction Quarterly* 1(3): 40-51.

Hill, D., L. E. Beutler, and R. Daldrup. 1989. "The Relationship of Process to Outcome in Brief Experiential Psychotherapy for Chronic Pain." *Journal of Clinical Psychology* 45(6): 951-57.

Hillman, J. and M. Ventura. 1992. *We've Had a Hundred Years of Psychotherapy—And the World's Getting Worse.* San Francisco: Harper.

Hoberman, H. M., P. M. Lewinsohn, and M. Tilson. 1988. "Group Treatment of Depression: Individual Predictors of Outcome." *Journal of Consulting and Clinical Psychology* 56(3): 393-98.

Hollister, W. G., J. W. Edgerton, and R. H. Hunter. 1985. *Alternative Services in Community Mental Health.* Chapel Hill: N.C.

Holroyd, K. A. and F. Andrasik. 1982. "Do the Effects of Cognitive Therapy Endure? A Two-Year Follow-up of Tension Headache Sufferers Treated with Cognitive Therapy or Biofeedback." *Cognitive Therapy and Research* 6(3): 325-34.

Holt, R. R. 1994. Letter in *New York Review of Books.* April 21, 66.

Holtzworth-Munroe, A., N. S. Jacobson, and M. Deklyen. 1989. "Relationship Between Behavioral Marital Therapy Outcome and Process Variables." *Journal of Consulting and Clinical Psychology* 57(5): 658-62.

Homer-Dixon, T. F., J. H. Buotwell, and G. W. Rathjens. 1993. "Environmental Change and Violent Conflict." *Scientific American* (February): 38-45.

Hook, S. 1959. *Psychoanalysis, Scientific Method, and Philosophy* New York: New York University Press.

Howard, K. I., S. M. Kopta, and M. S. Krause. 1986. "The Dose-effect Relationship in Psychotherapy." *American Psychologist* (February): 159-64.

Hsu, L. K. G. 1980. "Outcome of Anorexia Nervosa." *Archives of General Psychiatry* 37(September): 1041-46.

Huber, C. H. and B. Milstein. 1985. "Cognitive Restructuring and a Collaborative Set in Couples' Work." *American Journal of Family Therapy* 13(2): 17-27.

Imber, S. D., P. A. Pilkonis, S. M. Sotsky, I. Elkin, J. T. Watkins, J. F. Collins, M. T. Shea, W. R. Leber, and D. R. Glass. 1990. "Mode-Specific Effects Among Three Treatments for Depression." *Journal of Consulting and Clinical Psychology* 58(3): 352-59.

Iverson, A. and D. H. Baucom. 1990. "Behavioral Marital Therapy Outcomes: Alternate Interpretations of the Data." *Behavior Therapy* 21: 129-38.

Jacobson, N. S. 1984. "Component Analysis of Behavioral Marital Therapy: The Relative Effectiveness of Behavior Exchange and Communication/Problem-Solving Training." *Journal of Consulting and Clinical Psychology* 52(2): 295-305.

Jacobson, N. S., W. C. Follette, D. Revenstorf, D. H. Baucom, K. Hahlweg, and G. Margolin. 1984. "Variability in Outcome and Clinical Significance of Behavioral Marital Therapy: A Reanalysis of Outcome Data." *Journal of Consulting and Clinical Psychology* 52(4): 497-504.

———1989. "Research-Structured vs. Clinically Flexible Versions of Social Learning-Based Marital Therapy." *Behavioral Research and Therapy* 27(2): 173-80.

Jarrett, R. B. and R. O. Nelson. 1987. "Mechanisms of Change in Cognitive Therapy of Depression." *Behavior Therapy* 18:227-41.

Joanning, H. 1982. "The Long-Term Effects of the Couple Communication Program." *Journal of Marital and Family Therapy* (October): 463-68.
Johnson, S. M. and L. S. Greenberg. 1985. "Emotionally Focused Couples Therapy: An Outcome Study." *Journal of Marital and Family Therapy* 11(3): 313-17.
Kaminer, W. 1992. *I'm Dysfunctional; You're Dysfunctional.* Reading, Mass.: Addison-Wesley Publishing Company.
Kane, M. T. and P. C. Kendall. 1989. "Anxiety Disorders in Children: A Multiple-Baseline Evaluation of a Cognitive-Behavioral Treatment." *Behavior Therapy* 20: 499-508.
Kang, S., P. H. Kleinman, G. E. Woody, R. B. Millman, T. C. Todd, J. Kemp, and D. S. Lipton. 1991. "Outcomes for Cocaine Abusers After Once-a-Week Psychosocial Therapy." *American Journal of Psychiatry* 148(5): 630-35.
Kazdin, A. E., D. Bass, T. Siegel, and C. Thomas. 1989. "Cognitive-Behavioral Therapy and Relationship Therapy in the Treatment of Children Referred for Antisocial Behavior." *Journal of Consulting and Clinical Psychology* 57(4): 522-35.
Keane, T. M., J. A. Fairbank, and J. M. Caddell. 1989. "Implosive (Flooding) Therapy Reduces Symptoms of PTSD in Vietnam Veterans." *Behavior Therapy* 20: 245-60.
Kleinman, A. 1988. *Rethinking Psychiatry.* New York: The Free Press.
Klerman, G. L. 1983. "The Efficacy of Psychotherapy as the Basis for Public Policy." *The American Psychologist* (August):929-34.
———. 1986. "The Scientific Tasks Confronting Psychoanalysis." *The Behavior and Brain Sciences* 9(2): 245.
———. 1990. "The Psychiatric Patient's Rights to Effective Treatment: Implications of Osheroff v. Chestnut Lodge." *American Journal of Psychiatry* 147(4): 409-18.
Kline, P. 1988. *Psychology Exposed or the Emperor's New Clothes.* London: Routledge.
Klosko, J. S., D. H. Barlow, R. Tassinari, and J. A. Cerny. 1990. "A Comparison of Alprazolam and Behavior Therapy in Treatment of Panic Disorder." *Journal of Consulting and Clinical Psychology* 58(1): 77-84.
Kratochwill, T. R. 1978. *Single Subject Research.* New York: Academic Press.
Kurzweil, E. 1989. *The Freudians.* New Haven, Conn.: Yale University Press.
Lambert, M., F. D. Weber, and J. D. Sykes. 1993. "Psychotherapy versus Placebo Therapies: A review of the Metaanalytic Literature." Poster presented at the annual Meeting of the Western Psychological Association, Phoenix, Arizona, 1993.
Lambert, M. J. 1976. "Spontaneous Remission in Adult Neurotic Disorders: A Revision and Summary." *Psychological Bulletin* 83(1): 107-19.
Lambert, M. J. and A. E. Bergin. 1994. "The Effectiveness of Psychotherapy." In Bergin and Garfield (eds.). *Handbook of Psychotherapy and Behavior Change.* New York: John Wiley, 143-190.
Lambert, M. J., E. R. Christensen, and S. S. DeJulio. 1984. "The Assessment of Psychotherapy Outcome." In S. L. Garfield and A. E. Bergin (eds). *Handbook of Psychotherapy and Behavior Change.* New York: John Wiley, 23-62.
Lambert, M. J., D. A. Shapiro, and A. E. Bergin. 1986. "The Effectiveness of Psychotherapy." In S. L. Garfield and A. E. Bergin, editors. *Handbook of Psychotherapy and Behavior Change.* New York: John Wiley, 157-211.
Landman, J. T. and R. M. Dawes. 1982. "Psychotherapy Outcome: Smith and Glass' conclusions Stand Up Under Scrutiny." *American Psychologist* 37(5): 504-16.
Lash, S. (ed.). 1991. *Post-Structuralist and Post-Modernist Sociology.* Brookfield, Vt.: Edward Elgar Hopkins University Press.
Leff, J., L. Kuipers, R. Berkowitz, and D. Sturgeon. 1982. "A Controlled Trial of Social Intervention in the Families of Schizophrenic Patients." *British Journal of Psychiatry* 141: 121-34.

Lerman, P. 1975. *Community Treatment and Social Control: A critical Analysis of Juvenile Correctional Policy*. Chicago, Ill.: University of Chicago Press.

Lester, M. E. and W. J. Doherty. 1983. "Couples' Long-Term Evaluations of Their Marriage Encounter Experience." *Journal of Marital and Family Therapy* 9(2): 183-88.

Lewinsohn, P. M., G. N. Clarke, H. Hops, and J. Andrews. 1990. "Cognitive-Behavioral Treatment for Depressed Adolescents." *Behavior Therapy* 21: 385-401.

Lewontin, R. C. 1994. "Women vs. the Biologists." *The New York Review of Books*, April 7, 32.

Liddle, H. A. and R. J. Halpin. 1978. "Family Therapy Training and Supervision Literature: A Comparative Review." *Journal of Marriage and Family Counseling* 4: 77-98.

Lieberman, A. F., D. R. Weston, and J. H. Pawl. 1991. "Preventative Intervention and Outcome with Anxiously Attached Dyads." *Child Development* 62(1): 199-209.

Litt, M. D., T. F. Babor, F. K. DelBoca, R. M. Kadeen, and N. L. Cooney. 1992. "Types of Alcoholics, II: Application of an Empirically Derived Typology to Treatment Matching." *Archives of General Psychiatry* 49(8): 609-14.

Luborsky, L., B. Singer, and L. Luborsky. 1975. "Comparative Studies of Psychotherapies: Is It True that 'Everybody has Won and All Must have Prizes'?" *Archives of General Psychiatry* 32(August): 995-1008.

Malgady, R. G., L. H. Rogler, and G. Costantino. 1990. "Culturally Sensitive Psychotherapy for Puerto Rican Children and Adolescents: A Program of Treatment Outcome Research." *Journal of Consulting and Clinical Psychology* 58(6): 704-12.

Mann, B. J., C. M. Borduin, S. W. Henggeler, and D. M. Blaske. 1990. "An Investigation of Systemic Conceptualizations of Parent-Child Coalitions and Symptom Change." *Journal of Consulting and Clinical Psychology* 58(3): 336-44.

Manne, S. L., W. H. Redd, and P. B. Jacobsen. 1990. "Behavioral Intervention to Reduce Child and Parent Distress During Venipuncture." *Journal of Consulting and Clinical Psychology* 58(5): 565-72.

Marchione, K. E., L. Michelson, M. Greenwald, and C. Dancu. 1987. "Cognitive Behavioral Treatment of Agoraphobia." *Behavioral Research and Therapy* 255: 319-28. (Audio).

Marmar, C. R., L. Gaston, D. Gallagher, and L. W. Thompson. 1989. "Alliance and Outcome in Late-Life Depression." *Journal of Nervous and Mental Disease* 177(8): 464-72.

Martin, W. 1977. *The Kingdom of the Cults*. Minneapolis, Minn.: Bethany Fellowship.

Martinson, R. 1974. "What Works—Questions and Answers about Prison Reform." *Public Interest*. (Spring): 22-54.

Masson, J. 1988. *Against Therapy: Emotional Tyranny and the Myth of Psychological Healing*. New York: Atheneum.

Masten, A. S. 1979. "Family Therapy as a Treatment for Children: A Critical Review of Outcome Research." *Family Process* 18: 303-35.

Mattick, R. P. and L. Peters. 1988. "Treatment of Severe Social Phobia: Effects of Guided Exposure with and without Cognitive Restructuring." *Journal of Consulting and Clinical Psychology* 56(2): 251-60.

May, P. R. A. 1971. "For Better or Worse? Psychotherapy and Variance Change: A Critical Review of the Literature." *Journal of Nervous and Mental Disease* 152: 184-92.

Mays, D. T. and C. M. Franks. 1980. "Getting Worse: Psychotherapy or No Treatment—The Jury Should Still be Out." *Professional Psychology* 11: 78-92.

McCubbin, M. A. and H. I. McCubbin. In Figley, *Treating Family Stress*. New York: Bruner/Mazel Inc., 3-66.

McHugh, P. R. and P. R. Slavney. 1983. *The Perspectives of Psychiatry*. Baltimore: The Johns Hopkins University Press.

McLean, P. and S. Taylor. 1992. "Severity of Unipolar Depression and Choice of Treatment." *Behavioral Research and Therapy* 30(5): 443–51.

McLean, P. D. and A. R. Hakstian. 1990. "Relative Endurance of Unipolar Depression Treatment Effects: Longitudinal Follow-up." *Journal of Consulting and Clinical Psychology* 58(4): 482–88.

Mehlman, S. K., D. H. Baucom, and D. Anderson. 1983. "Effectiveness of Co-Therapists Versus Single Therapists and Immediate Versus Delayed Treatment in Behavioral Marital Therapy." *Journal of Consulting and Clinical Psychology* 51(2): 258–66.

Melin, L. and S. J. Linton. 1988. "A Follow-Up Study of a Comprehensive Behavioural Treatment Programme for Chronic Pain Patients." *Behavioural Psychotherapy* 16(4): 313–21.

Meltzoff, J. and M. Kornreich. 1970. *Research in Psychotherapy*. New York: Atherton.

Meyer, J. and B. Rowan. 1977. "Institutionalized Organizations: Formal Structure as Myth and Ceremony." *American Journal of Sociology* 83(2): 340–63.

Miller, I. W., W. H. Norman, G. I. Keitner, S. B. Bishop, and M. G. Dow. 1989. "Cognitive-Behavioral Treatment of Depressed Inpatients." *Behavior Therapy* 20: 25–47.

Miller, R. C. and J. S. Berman. 1983. "The Efficacy of Cognitive Behavior Therapies: A Quantitative Review of the Research Evidence." *Psychological Bulletin* 94(1): 39–53.

Miller S., E. W. Nunnally, and D. Wackman. "Minnesota Couples Communication Program (MCCP): Premarital and Marital Groups." In D. H. L. Olson (ed.). *Treating Relationships*. 1976. Lake Mills, Iowa: Graphic Publishing Co.

Miller, W. R. 1980. "Focused Versus Broad-Spectrum Behavior Therapy for Problem Drinkers." *Journal of Consulting and Clinical Psychology* 48(5): 590–601.

Mitchell, J. E., R. L. Pyle, E. D. Eckert, D. Hatsukami, C. Pomeroy, R. Zimmerman. 1990. "A Comparison Study of Antidepressants and Structured Intensive Group Psychotherapy in the Treatment of Bulimia Nervosa." *Archives of General Psychiatry* 47(February): 149–57.

Morris, J. B. 1987. "Group Psychotherapy for Prolonged Postnatal Depression." *British Journal of Medical Psychology* 60: 279–81.

Nagel, T. 1994. "Freud's Permanent Revolution." *New York Review of Books*, May 12, 34–38.

Neimeyer, R. A. and G. Feixas. 1990. "The Role of Homework and Skill Acquisition in the Outcome of Group cognitive Therapy for Depression." *Behavior Therapy* 21(3): 281–92.

New York Review. 1994. Letters (Responses to "The Unknown Freud") 31(3): 34–44.

Nezu, A. M. and M. G. Perri. 1989. "Social Problem-Solving Therapy for Unipolar Depression: An Initial Dismantling Investigation." *Journal of Consulting and Clinical Psychology* 57(3): 408–13.

Nichols, M. P. and R. C. Schwartz. 1991. *Family Therapy*. Needham Heights, Mass.: Allyn and Bacon.

Norris, C. 1990. *What's Wrong with Postmodernism*. Baltimore, Md.: Johns Hopkins University Press.

O'Farrell, T. J., H. S. Cutter, and F. J. Floyd. 1985. "Evaluating Behavioral Marital Therapy for Male Alcoholics: Effects on Marital Adjustment and Communication from Before to After Treatment." *Behavior Therapy* 16: 147–67.

Office of Technology Assessment. 1980. "The Implications of Cost-Effectiveness Analysis of Medical Technology." Background Paper #3: The Efficacy and Cost Effectiveness of Psychotherapy. United States Congress: Washington, D.C.

O'Leary, K. D. 1981. "A Comparative Outcome Study of Behavioral Marital Therapy and Communication Therapy." *Journal of Marital and Family Therapy* 7: 159-69.

O'Leary, K. D. and S. R. H. Beach. 1990. "Marital Therapy: A Viable Treatment for Depression and Marital Discord." *American Journal of Psychiatry* 147(2): 183-86.

Olmstead, M. P., R. Dais, W. Rockert, M. J. Irvine, M. Eagle, and D. M. Garner. 1991. "Efficacy of a Brief Group Psychoeducational Intervention for Bulimia Nervosa." *Behavior Research and Therapy* 29(1): 71-83.

Olson, D. H., C. S. Russell, and D. H. Sprenkle. 1980. "Marital and Family Therapy: A Decade Review." *Journal of Marriage and the Family* 42: 973-94.

Pallone, N. J. 1986. *On the Social Utility of Psychotherapy*. New Brunswick, N. J.: Transaction Publishers.

Palmer, T. 1974. "The Youth Authority's Community Treatment Program." *Federal Probation* 38(1): 3-14.

Parloff, M. B. 1978. *Assessment of Psychosocial Treatment of Mental Health Disorders: Current Status and Prospects*. Rockville, Md.: Clinical Research Branch, National Institute of Mental Health.

Patterson, C. H. 1984. "Empathy, Warmth, and Genuineness in Psychotherapy: A Review of Reviews." *Psychotherapy* 21(4): 431-38.

Persons, J. B. 1991. "Psychotherapy Outcome Studies Do Not Accurately Represent Current Models of Psychotherapy." *American Psychologist*. February 46(2): 99-106.

Piel, G. 1993. (Book review). "Can History Stop Repeating Itself?" *Preparing for the Twenty First Century* by Paul Kennedy. *Scientific American* 269(1-July): 114-17.

Pilkonis, P. A., S. D. Imber, P. Lewis, and P. Rubinsky. 1984. "A Comparative Outcome Study of Individual, Group, and Conjoint Psychotherapy." *Archives of General Psychiatry* 41(May): 431-37.

Piper, W. E., H. F. Azim, M. McCallum, and A. S. Joyce. 1990. "Patient Suitability and Outcome in Short-Term Individual Psychotherapy." *Journal of Consulting and Clinical Psychology* 58(4): 475-81.

Pisterman, S., P. J. McGrath, and P. Firestone. 1989. "Outcome of Parent-Mediated Treatment of Preschoolers with Attention Deficit Disorder with Hyperactivity." *Journal of Consulting and Clinical Psychology* 57(5): 628-35.

Polsky, A. J. 1991. *The Rise of the Therapeutic State*. Princeton, N. J.: Princeton University Press.

Popenoe, D. 1993. "Scholars Should Worry About the Disintegration of the American Family." *Chronicle of Higher Education*. April 14: A48.

Pra, M. 1971. "For Better or for Worse? Psychotherapy and Variance Change: A Critical Review of the Literature." *Journal of Nervous and Mental Disease* 152: 184-92.

Prioleau, L., M. Murdock, and N. Brody. 1983. "An Analysis of Psychotherapy Versus Placebo Studies." *Behavioral and Brain Sciences* 6: 275-310.

Pyle, R., J. E. Mitchell, E. D. Eckert, D. Hatsukami, C. Pomeroy, and R. Zimmerman. 1990. "Maintenance Treatment and 6-Month Outcome for Bulimic Patients Who Respond to Initial Treatment." *American Journal of Psychiatry* 147(7): 871-75.

Rachman, S. 1971. *The Effects of Psychological Treatment*. Oxford: Perragon Press.

Rachman, S. J. and G. T. Wilson. 1980. *The Effects of Psychological Therapy*. New York: Pergamon Press.

Raue, J. and S. H. Spence. 1985. "Group versus Individual Applications of Reciprocity Training for Parent-Youth Conflict." *Behaviour Research and Therapy* 23(2): 177-86.

Ravetz, R. R. 1979. *Scientific Knowledge and Its Social Problems*. New York: Oxford University Press.

———. 1990. *The Merger of Knowledge with Power*. London and New York: Mansell Publishing Limited.

Raz-Duvshani, A. 1986. "Cognitive Structure Changes with Psychotherapy in Neurosis." *British Journal of Medical Psychology* 59: 341–50.

Reid, W. J. and P. Hanrahan. 1982. "Recent Evaluations of Social Work: Grounds for Optimism." *Social Work* 27(4): 328–40.

Rehm, L. P., S. J. Kornblith, M. W. O'Hara, D. M. Lamparski, J. M. Romano, and J. I. Volkin. 1981. "An Evaluation of Major Components in a Self-Control Therapy Program for Depression." *Behavior Modification* 5(4): 459–89.

———. 1987. "Cognitive and Behavioral Targets in a Self-Control Therapy Program for Depression." *Journal of Consulting and Clinical Psychology* 55(1): 60–67.

Resick, P. A., C. G. Jordan, S. A. Girelli, C. K. Hutter, and S. Marhoefe. 1988. "A Comparative Outcome Study of Behavioral Group Therapy for Sexual Assault Victims." *Behavior Therapy* 19(3): 385–401.

Rieff, P. 1966. *The Triumph of the Therapeutic*. New York: Harper and Row.

Roazen, P. 1990. *Encountering Freud*. New Brunswick, N. J.: Transaction Publishers.

Rosen, G. 1968. *Madness in Society*. Chicago: University of Chicago Press.

Rosenau, P. M. 1992. *Post-modernism and the Social Sciences*. Princeton, N. J.: Princeton University Press.

Rosenthal, R. 1983. "Assessing the Statistical and Social Importance of the Effects of Psychotherapy." *Journal of Consulting and Clinical Psychology* 51(1): 4–13.

Rosenthal, R. and D. B. Rubin. 1978. "Interpersonal Expectancy Effects: The First 345 Studies." *Behavioral and Brain Sciences* 3: 377–415.

Rounsaville, B. J., E. S. Chevron, B. A. Prusoff, I. Elkin, S. Imber, S. Sotsky, and J. Watkins. 1987. "The Relation Between Specific and General Dimensions of the Psychotherapy Process in Interpersonal Psychotherapy of Depression." *Journal of Consulting and Clinical Psychology* 55(3): 379–84.

Roustang, F. 1980. *Psychoanalysis Never Lets Go*. Baltimore, Md.: The Johns Hopkins University Press.

Russell, C. S., R. B. Atilano, S. A. Anderson, A. P. Jurich, and L. P. Bergen. 1984. "Intervention Strategies: Predicting Family Therapy Outcome." *Journal of Marital and Family Therapy* 10(3): 241–51.

Russell, G. F. M., G. I. Szmukler, C. Dare, and I. Eisler. 1987. "An Evaluation of Family Therapy in Anorexia Nervosa and Bulimia Nervosa." *Archives of General Psychiatry* 44(December): 1047–56.

Saarijarvi, S., U. Rytokoski, and E. Alanen. 1991. "A Controlled Study of Couple Therapy in Chronic Low Back Pain Patients: No Improvement of Disability." *Journal of Psychosomatic Research* 35(6): 671–77.

Saarijarvi, S., E. Alanen, U. Rytokoski, and M. T. Hyyppa. 1992. "Couple Therapy Improves Mental Well-Being in Chronic Low Back Pain Patients: A Controlled, Five Year Follow-Up Study." *Journal of Psychosomatic Research* 36(7): 651–56.

Sannibale, C. 1989. "A Prospective Study of Treatment Outcome with a Group of Male Problem Drinkers." *Journal of Studies on Alcohol* 50(3): 236–44.

Sarup, M. 1989. *An Introductory Guide to Post-structuralism and Postmodernism*. Athens, Georgia: University of Georgia Press.

Sayger, T. V., S. A. Szykula, and C. Sudweeks. 1992. "Treatment Side Effects: Maternal Positive and Negative Attributes of Child-focused Family Therapy." *Child and Family Behavior Therapy* 14(1): 1–9.

Schofield, W. 1964. *Psychotherapy: The Purchase of Friendship*. Englewood Cliffs, N. J.: Prentice-Hall.

Schorske, W. E. 1993. (Book review.) "Freud's Egyptian Dig." *New York Review of Books*, May 27.

Schuerman, J. R., T. L. Rzepnicki, J. H. Littell, and A. Clark. 1993. *Evaluation of the Illinois Family First Placement Prevention Program: Final Report.* Illinois Department of Children and Family Services.

Schuerman, J. R., T. L. Rzepnicki, and J. H. Littell. 1994. *Putting Families First.* Hawthorne, New York: Aldine de Gruyter.

Schulte, D., R. Kunzel, G. Pepping, and T. Schulte-Bahrenberg. 1992. "Tailor-made Versus Standardized Therapy of Phobic Patients." *Advances in Behavior Research and Therapy* 14: 67-92.

Scogin, F., C. Jamison, and K. Gochneaur. 1989. "Comparative Efficacy of Cognitive and Behavioral Bibliotherapy for Mildly and Moderately Depressed Older Adults." *Journal of Consulting and Clinical Psychology* 57(3): 403-07.

Sechrest, L., S. O. White, and E. D. Brown (eds.). 1979. *The Rehabilitation of Criminal Offenders.* Washington, D.C.: National Academy of Sciences.

Seidman, S. and D. G. Wagner (eds.). 1992. *Postmodernism and Social Theory.* Cambridge, Mass.: Blackwell.

Senediak, C. and S. H. Spence. 1985. "Rapid versus Gradual Scheduling of Therapeutic Contact in a Family Based Behavioural Weight Control Programme for Children." *Behavioural Psychotherapy* 13(4): 265-87.

Shapiro, D. A. 1985. "Recent Applications of Meta-analyses in Clinical Research." *Clinical Psychology Review* 5: 13-34.

Shapiro, D. A., M. Barkham, G. E. Hardy, and L. A. Morrison. 1990. "The Second Sheffield Psychotherapy Project: Rationale, Design and Preliminary Outcome Data." *British Journal of Medical Psychology* 63: 97-108.

Shapiro, D. A. and D. Shapiro. 1983. "Comparative Therapy Outcome Research: Methodological Implications of Meta-Analysis." *Journal of Consulting and Clinical Psychology* 51(1): 42-53.

———. 1982a. "Meta-Analysis of Comparative Therapy Outcome Research: A Critical Review." *Behavioral Psychotherapy* 10: 4-25.

———. 1982b. "Meta-Analysis of Comparative Therapy Outcome Studies: A Republication and Refinement." *Psychological Bulletin* 93(3): 581-604.

Shipley, R. H. and P. A. Boudewyns. 1980. "Flooding and Implosive Therapy: Are They Harmful?" *Behavior Therapy* 11: 503-08.

Sigrell, B., 1992. "The Long-term Effects of Group Psychotherapy: A Thirteen-Year Follow-up Study." *Group Analysis* 25: 333-52.

Silverman, J. S., J. A. Silverman, and D. A. Eardley. 1984. "Do Maladaptive Attitudes Cause Depression?" *Archives of General Psychiatry* 41(January): 28-30.

Silverman, W. 1991. "Person's Description of Psychotherapy Outcome Studies Does Not Accurately Represent Psychotherapy Outcome Studies." *American Psychologist* (December): 1351-52.

Simons, A. D., G. E. Murphy, J. L. Levine, and R. D. Wetzel. 1986. "Cognitive Therapy and Pharmacotherapy for Depression." *Archives of General Psychiatry* 43(January): 43-48.

Smith, M. L. and G. V. Glass. 1977. "Meta-Analysis of Psychotherapy Outcome Studies." *American Psychologist* 32(September): 752-60.

Smith, M. L., G. V. Glass, and T. I. Miller. 1980. *The Benefits of Psychotherapy.* Baltimore Md.: Johns Hopkins Press.

Smith, S. R. and M. Lipsky. 1993. *Nonprofits for Hire: The Welfare State in the Age of Contracting.* Cambridge, Mass.: Harvard University Press.

Smith, T. E., S. P. Sells, and N. Newfield (unpublished). "Evaluating Ethnographies in Family Therapy Using Methodological Goodness Criteria.

Snyder, D. K. and R. M. Wills. 1989. "Behavioral Versus Insight-Oriented Marital Therapy: Effects on Individual and Interpersonal Functioning." *Journal of Consulting and Clinical Psychology* 57(1): 39-46.

Snyder, D. K., R. M. Wills, and A. Grady-Fletcher. 1991. "Long-Term Effectiveness of Behavioral Versus Insight-Oriented Marital Therapy: A 4-Year Follow-Up Study." *Journal of Consulting and Clinical Psychology* 59(1): 138-41.

Sokol, L., A. T. Beck, R. L. Greenberg, F. D. Wright, and R. J. Berchick. 1989. "Cognitive Therapy of Panic Disorder." *Journal of Nervous and Mental Disease* 177(12-December): 711-16.

Sotsky, S. M., D. R. Glass, T. Shea, P. A. Pilkonis, J. F. Collins, I. Elkin, J. T. Watkins, S. D. Imber, W. R. Leber, J. Moyer, and M. E. Oliveri. 1991. "Patient Predictors of Response to Psychotherapy and Pharmacotherapy: Findings in the NIMH Treatment of Depression Collaborative Research Program." *American Journal of Psychiatry* 148(8): 997-1008.

Specht, H. 1990. "Social Work and the Popular Psychotherapies." *Social Service Review* (September): 345-57.

Specht, H. and M. Courtney. 1993. *Unfaithful Angels*. New York: Free Press.

Sprenkle, D. H. and C. L. Storm. 1983. "Divorce Therapy Outcome Research: A Substantive and Methodological Review." *Journal of Marital and Family Therapy* 9(3): 239-58.

Stanton, A. H., J. G. Gunderson, P. H. Knapp, A. F. Frank, M. L. Vannicelli, R. Schnitzer, and R. Rosenthal. 1984. "Effects of Psychotherapy in Schizophrenia, I: Design and Implementation of a Controlled Study." *Schizophrenia Bulletin* 10: 520-63.

Stanton, M. D. 1979. "Family Treatment Approaches to Drug Abuse Problems: A Review." *Family Process* 18: 251-80.

Stanton, M. D., F. Steier, and T. C. Todd. 1982. "Paying Families for Attending Sessions: Counteracting the Dropout Problem." *Journal of Marital and Family Therapy* 8: 371-73.

Stein, L. I., and M. A. Test. 1980. "Alternatives to Mental Hospital Treatment." *Archives of General Psychiatry* 37(April): 392-412.

Steinbrueck, S. M., S. E. Maxwell, and G. S. Howard. 1983. "A Meta-Analysis of Psychotherapy and Drug Therapy in the Treatment of Unipolar Depression with Adults." *Journal of Consulting and Clinical Psychology* 51(6): 856-63.

Strube, M. J. and D. P. Hartmann. 1982. "A Critical Appraisal of Meta-Analysis." *British Journal of Clinical Psychology* 21: 129-39.

———. 1983. "Meta-Analysis: Techniques, Applications, and Functions." *Journal of Consulting and Clinical Psychology* 51(1): 14-27.

Swift, W. J. 1982. "The Long-Term Outcome of Early Onset Anorexia Nervosa." *Journal of the American Academy of Child Psychiatry* 21: 38-46.

Szapocznik, J., W. M. Kurtines, F. H. Foote, A. Perez-Vidal, and O. Hervis. 1983. "Conjoint Versus One-Person Family Therapy: Some Evidence for the Effectiveness of Conducting Family Therapy Through One Person." *Journal of Consulting and Clinical Psychology* 51(6): 889-99.

Szapocznik, J., E. Murray, M. Scopetta, O. Hervis, A. Rio, R. Cohen, A. Rivas-Vazquez, V. Posada, and W. Kurtines. 1989. "Structural Family Versus Psychodynamic Child Therapy for Problematic Hispanic Boys." *Journal of Consulting and Clinical Psychology* 57(5): 571-78.

Szasz, T. 1965. *The Ethics of Psychoanalysis*. New York: Basic Books.

———. 1978. *The Myth of Psychotherapy*. Garden City, N.Y.: Anchor Press.

———. 1984. *The Therapeutic State*. Buffalo, N.Y.: Prometheus.

Telch, C. F., W. S. Agras, and E. M. Rossiter. 1990. "Group Cognitive-Behavioral Treatment for the Nonpurging Bulimic: An Initial Evaluation." *Journal of Consulting and Clinical Psychology* 58(5): 629–35.

Thompson, L. W., D. Gallagher, and J. S. Breckenridge. 1987. "Comparative Effectiveness of Psychotherapies for Depressed Elders." *Journal of Consulting and Clinical Psychology* 55(3): 385–90.

Tillitski, C. J. 1990. "A Meta-Analysis of Estimated Effect Sizes for Group versus Individual versus Control Treatments." *International Journal of Group Psychotherapy* 40(2): 215–24.

Torrey, E. F. 1986. *Witchdoctors and Psychiatrists: The Common Roots of Psychotherapy and its Future*. New York: Harper and Row.

Tosi, D. J., D. R. Rudy, J. Lewis, and M. A. Murphy. 1992. "The Psychobiological Effects of Cognitive Experiential Therapy, Hypnosis, Cognitive Restructuring, and Attention Placebo Control in the Treatment of Essential Hypertension." *Psychotherapy* 29(2): 274–84.

Truax, C. B., and R. R. Carkhuff. 1967. *Toward Effective Counseling and Psychotherapy: Training and Practice*. Chicago: Aldine Publishing Co.

Vattimo, G. 1988. *The End of Modernity*. Baltimore: The Johns Hopkins University Press.

Wampler, K. S. 1982a. "The Effectiveness of the Minnesota Couple Communication Program: A Review of Research." *Journal of Marital and Family Therapy* 8: 345–56.

———. 1982b. "Bringing the Review of Literature into the Age of Quantification: Meta-Analysis as a Strategy for Integrating Research Findings in Family Studies." *Journal of Marriage and the Family* 44: 1009–23.

Waring, E. M., C. A. Stalker, C. M. Carver, and M. Z. Gitta. 1991. "Waiting List Controlled Trial of Cognitive Marital Therapy in Severe Marital Discord." *Journal of Marital and Family Therapy* 17(3): 243–56.

Waring, E. M., C. Carver, C. A. Stalker, R. Fry, and B. Schaefer. 1990. "A Randomized Clinical Trial of Cognitive Marital Therapy." *Journal of Sex and Marital Therapy* 16(3): 165–80.

Weinstein, M. 1988. "Preparation of Children for Psychotherapy Through Videotaped Modeling." *Journal of Clinical Child Psychology* 17(2): 131–36.

Weisz, J. R., B. Weiss, M. D. Alicke, and M. L. Klotz. 1987. "Effectiveness of Psychotherapy with Children and Adolescents: A Meta-Analysis for Clinicians." *Journal of Consulting and Clinical Psychology* 55: 542–49.

Weisz, J. R., B. R. Walter, B. Weiss, G. A. Fernandez, and V. A. Mikow. 1990. "Arrests among Emotionally Disturbed Violent and Assaultive Individuals Following Minimal Versus Lengthy Intervention Through North Carolina's Willie M Program." *Journal of Consulting and Clinical Psychology* 58(6): 720–28.

Wellisch, D. K. and G. K. Ro-Trock. 1980. "A Three-Year Follow-up of Family Therapy." *International Journal of Family Therapy* 2(3): 169–75.

Wells, R. A. and A. E. Dezen. 1978. "The Results of Family Therapy Revisited: The Nonbehavioral Methods." *Family Process* 17: 251–74.

Wetzel, R. D., G. E. Murphy, R. M. Carney, P. Whitworth, and M. A. Knesevic. 1992. "Prescribing Therapy for Depression: The Role of Learned Resourcefulness: A Failure to Replicate." *Psychological Reports* 70(3 Pt 1): 803–07.

Whitlatch, C. J., S. H. Zarit, and A. Von Eye. 1991. "Efficacy of Interventions with Caregivers: A Reanalysis." *Gerontologist* 31(1): 9–14.

Williams, S. L., P. J. Kinney, and J. Falbo. 1989. "Generalization of Therapeutic Changes in Agoraphobia: The Role of Perceived Self-Efficacy." *Journal of Consulting and Clinical Psychology* 57(3): 436–42.

Winston, A., J. Pollack, L. McCullough, W. Flegenheimer, R. Kestenbaum, and M. Trujillo. 1991. "Brief Psychotherapy of Personality Disorders." *Journal of Nervous and Mental Disease* 179(4): 188–93.

Woody, G. E., A. T. McLellan, and L. Luborsky. 1987. "Twelve-Month Follow-Up of Psychotherapy for Opiate Dependence." *American Journal of Psychiatry* 144(5-May): 590–96.

Wootton, B. 1959. *Social Science and Social Pathology.* London: George Allen and Unwin.

Yohman, J. R., K. W. Schaeffer, and O. A. Parsons. 1988. "Cognitive Training in Alcoholic Men." *Journal of Consulting and Clinical Psychology* 56(1): 67–72.

Zweben, A., S. Pearlman, and S. Li. 1988. "A Comparison of Brief Advice and Conjoint Therapy in the Treatment of Alcohol Abuse: The Results of the Marital Systems Study." *British Journal of Addiction* 83(8): 899–916.

Index

Made in the USA
Monee, IL
13 September 2026

62976815R00109